Over 50, Overweight & Out of Breath!

Over 50, Overweight & Out of Breath

A Year of Going from
Super Fat to Super Fit

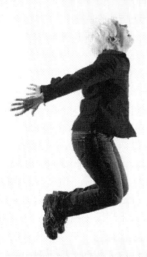

Laura E. Sinclair

Book cover and interior design by Jean Boles
http://jeanboles.elance.com

*This book is dedicated to my
loving partner, Linda.*

Contents

Chapter One: *Change Agent*

"There are no short cuts to anyplace worth going." —Beverly Sills

I remember back in the 60s, I was watching an episode of the classic television show, "The Beverly Hillbillies." Granny had convinced banker, Milburn Drysdale, that she had a cure for the common cold. Mr. Drysdale saw this as a golden opportunity to make millions of dollars for himself and his bank. He went ahead with plans to market this amazing elixir, all the while trying to get Granny to reveal her secret recipe. Finally, after much nagging and persistence, she told him her secret cure for the common cold. She held up her jug of moonshine and said, "Take a few sips of this every day for seven days and you will be cured!"

We all know that after seven days of experiencing a cold, we are either all better or almost there. The point of this story is that so far there is no cure for the common cold; there is also no secret to losing weight and keeping it off. It is the same as it has always been: eat less and move more. How you go about doing these two things is the difference between losing weight and becoming super fit. I will share in the following pages the story of how I lost more than 80 pounds in just over a year—and why. The why part of the story is just as interesting to me as the actual weight loss. Why, at 55 years old, did I decide to lose the weight I had gained over a 12-year period? What was the motivation for making this decision?

In the year of my weight loss, I went from being *morbidly obese*, to obese, to overweight, to normal weight, and presently, to being at a level of fitness that has exceeded my wildest dreams.

In July of 2011 I broke my leg in three places—what is known as a trimalleolar fracture. This turned out to be a major catalyst for deciding to make massive changes in my life, starting with losing the weight. I had been overweight for years, but this event led to a multitude of experiences that gave me insight and understanding into what it was like to be physically handicapped. I was lucky that it was a temporary condition.

The year before I broke my leg I had wanted to make big changes, but life got in the way. I asked for change and the universe delivered big time. I look at breaking my leg as symbolic of breaking with my past life and beginning anew. Life is a series of choices, and I decided to make some new ones. The first one was to lose all of the weight and keep it off this time. How I went about achieving this goal is what I refer to as my *triple combo of success*. The three components to my success—which I will detail later—are equally important. These components go hand in hand and were the perfect formula for my successful weight loss.

A funny thing happened as my motivation for losing weight evolved over the year. My initial reason for losing weight began with my accident, but over time, it became bigger than that. The leg break was the catalyst

to seeing the bigger picture of my life at age 55. My reasons for losing weight had less to do with vanity (still very important) and more to do with taking control of my overall health so that I could give myself the best chance of having a healthy and lengthy aging process.

If you are reading this book chances are you are over 50 years old. If you are younger and in good health, you will eventually pass the 50-year mark—trust me. Everyone is surprised when they get there. I am a member of the baby boomer generation. Baby boomers are those folks who were born from 1946 through 1964. Currently, there are 78 million of us alive. I happen to fall in the middle, being born in 1955. As a group, we are considered to be the wealthiest, most active and physically fit generation up to this time. In 2011, the first of the baby boomers reached the retirement age of 65. During the next eighteen years boomers will turn 65 at the rate of 10,000 per day. The repercussions of 10,000 people entering retirement each day will be felt for years to come, especially in the area of health care. I believe it is our responsibility to take ownership and lead a healthy lifestyle. Taking better care of ourselves by eating properly, not smoking, getting regular exercise and sleeping enough will put us all in a better position to stay healthy as we age. There is no denying that our environment, genetic code and a lot of luck also figure into a long life. However, doing our part to try to avoid chronic illness will certainly increase our chances of living a long and healthy life.

Baby boomers were the first generation to become fitness enthusiasts. This is a legacy that we proudly leave to the generations following ours. My grandmother never had a thought about running a marathon. It wasn't in her DNA to make time for exercise. That's not because she was lazy. She grew up on a farm in Nova Scotia. The fitness level of farmers in her day easily exceeded most of today's amateur athletes.

Thanks to advances in technology and medicine we are living longer. I was riding into Boston one evening and spotted a billboard that showed the following statement, "One in three people born today will live to be 100 years old." That is a long time, folks, and the benefits of living longer present challenges that we are just beginning to comprehend. The flip side of living longer is that the benefits of technology have taken the need for a lot of physical energy right out of the picture. Instead of living the hard, physically demanding farm life of my grandmother's time, we can do most everything sitting on our rear ends watching television, clicking a mouse or tapping the screen of our smart phone or tablet. Don't get me wrong. I love technology and most everything it has to offer, but if I didn't make time to work out every day, the only part of my body that would be flexible and strong would be my index fingers. Sitting is not good for a human body that was built to move. The average adult spends 50 to 70 percent of their time sitting. As a freelance photojournalist, I used to spend hours editing and captioning pictures before uploading them to a folder on the Internet for publication. I would have my laptop perched on my lap for so long my legs would fall asleep. I often referred to this jokingly as computer legs. It was no joke. Now after I spend 30 minutes in front of the computer I get up and move around for at least a few minutes. I may do something as mundane as vacuum or just walking around doing anything other than sitting. I often stand and work at my computer. It sounds almost silly, but I need to do this type of activity, and now it is one of the personal tools that I use daily.

Once we turn 50 our metabolism slows down and we lose muscle tissue as well as bone mass. The structure that supports our bodies slowly deteriorates once we pass the 50-year mark. That's the bad news. The fantastic news is that we can slow this process down through good nutrition and workout programs that include cardio and strength training, using barbells and free weights. Dr. Jonathon Sullivan, an emergency room physician at the Detroit Receiving Hospital, wrote an excellent paper, "Barbell Training is Big Medicine". [1] Dr. Sullivan argues that using barbells to perform squats, bench presses and dead lifts sends a signal to the body to produce new muscle tissue, bone matrix and promote new cell growth. I buy into this 100 percent because I am living proof that it works.

Dr. Sullivan also states that using barbells for strength training is a form of medicine or a drug that you administer yourself. He posits that it is the only drug that you can safely increase the dose as you get stronger and healthier. There is something very empowering about this concept. As I mentioned earlier, we are living longer. This is a critical point. I realized when I broke my leg and was 80 pounds overweight that I had a choice of which path I would take for the next part of my life. I could continue along the same path of remaining *morbidly obese* and setting myself up for potential chronic illnesses such as Type II diabetes, heart disease, stroke or some form of cancer. Or, I could choose the other path. The other path would be a complete change in lifestyle where I would lose the weight, keep it off and become super fit. Happily, I chose the latter. I also decided to take it very slowly; it would be a marathon instead of a sprint. In other words, there would be no quick-fix diets or diving into a workout program that would be too much for me to handle in the beginning. I took baby steps all the way.

I belong to the speaking group, Toastmasters. One week I gave a speech about my year of getting fit. There was a guest in the audience who came up to me following my speech and asked if I had a photo of myself before I lost the 80 plus pounds. He said I didn't look like someone who had lost a lot of weight. That instead, I looked incredibly fit. I took this to be a great compliment. It was my intention from the start of my weight-loss journey to not be "skinny fat" but to become super fit. I have muscles, a strong and efficient heart and my metabolism is up. I do a lot of weight lifting, which results in an "after burn." What is an after burn? It is the time following a weight-lifting workout when your metabolism is running higher than normal, causing your body to burn more calories. Having a strong and fit body is empowering. I love the feeling of strength, and being strong affects every aspect of my daily activities. I even walk more confidently.

Barbells and free weights are powerful tools. I am not talking about a dainty workout for toning. Women can and should lift the same way men do. Women may not be able to lift the same amount of weight, but pushing ourselves hard regularly will pay dividends for years to come. According to Dr. Sullivan, if you can lift, you should, no matter what age. This includes people who are in their 60s, 70s and up. Strength training builds our muscles and makes our bodies strong. A strong and fit body is what we need more than ever as we age.

If someone had told me on July 3, 2011, the day after I broke my leg, that in little more than 12 months I would be 80 pounds lighter and reach a level of fitness that I never thought possible, I wouldn't have believed it. Of course, I was on powerful pain meds and my right leg was double the size of my left leg, so I could be forgiven for not seeing clearly into my crystal ball. I always say to people, "If I can do it anybody can!" And I mean it!

I am constantly changing. I change the food and the time that I eat it. I change the content of my workouts. I constantly try to initiate change into some aspect of my life every day. Why? When behavior becomes routine, we adapt physically and mentally. We become stale and uninteresting. I do not want to be stale and uninteresting. Time is short these days. Sometimes I catch myself asking where did the last 30 or 40 years go? This question serves as a great motivator to make every minute count. I am now giving myself the best chance at healthy aging, compressing that tiny sliver of time when my health fails and I leave the planet. This is not sad, or morbid; it is realistic. News flash: We are all going to die someday. We have no say when this is going to happen, but we can put ourselves in position to have the best, most healthy aging process by protecting and maintaining the vehicle—our body—that carries us through life.

I recently had a conversation with a friend. He made a comment about how I was "fading away" because I looked so thin. I said that I had not felt this good or been this fit in years. Also, I was surprised at the resiliency of the human body when given a chance to live an optimal lifestyle. This guy is a few years younger than me and has a huge gut and is heading down the path of unhealthy aging, meaning a heart attack or worse might be on the horizon for him. He responded by saying, "I know I could get in really great shape, but I just don't want to do the work." I found this surprising and sad. He has so little self-worth that he is tossing his health up in the air of uncertainty. In other words, he is playing Russian roulette with his life. I am not judging him. I was where he is for years. People have to reach their own break point. He may decide, "Yes, I am worth it," and make some great changes. It has to come from him and be his idea.

My life today is far different from two years ago. I zip upstairs and have tons more energy. I accomplish a lot more during my day. My skin is healthier. I no longer look away from my reflection. I get on a scale willingly and often. My knees and back no longer ache. I have rock-hard abs. I have muscle definition in my arms and back. I am super strong. I can bench press my weight. I am no longer embarrassed to walk into a room full of strangers because of feeling self-conscious about my weight. I have pride in myself and how I dress. I do not wear mom jeans. I never thought I would wear skinny jeans, but I do now. I was so unaccustomed to shopping that the salesperson brought in some size 6 jeans along with some size 8s. I was leaning toward the 8s when she asked, "Why wear size 8 when you can wear 6?" She was right, of course, but I was just getting my head around wearing jeans, never mind skinny jeans. Sometimes your mind takes a little longer to catch up with your physical changes. I am no longer the short, fat girl. I am healthy, powerful and more able to meet the challenges of being in my 50s and beyond.

Chances are you picked this book up because the title "Over 50, Overweight & Out of Breath" resonated with you. The subtitle "A Year of Going from Super Fat to Super Fit" grabbed your attention because it tapped into the far reaches of your mind. The title may have gotten you thinking about the potential and possibilities of changing your middle-aged body from soft and deteriorating to super fit with sculpted muscles and boundless energy. When I created the title the passing grade for success had to be, would I want to read this book? And the answer was a resounding yes. This is because before I wrote this book I was diagnosed as *morbidly obese* by my primary-care physician following a yearly visit. The only problem with this diagnosis was that we never discussed this issue. I knew I was very overweight, but it wasn't until I switched doctors and picked up my medical records that I saw this in writing. I have read that doctors do not feel comfortable telling their patients they are overweight. I saw myself in front of the mirror every day so I knew that things were bad, but it wasn't until I read those words—*morbidly obese*—that the gravity of the situation sunk in, but...not enough for me to get my act together right away and do something about it. It took a life-changing event, not a life-threatening event, but breaking my leg in all likelihood saved my life and most definitely improved the quality of my life. I was five feet and one inch tall. I weighed in at 190 pounds. There, I said it! I never thought about the actual number on the scale, but I do now. I am vain and being overweight depressed me, but now I was 55 and the stakes were higher. Sure, I wanted to look good again, but now there was the issue of staving off chronic illnesses that are associated with aging. Being *morbidly obese*— which means being 80-100 pounds or more over your normal weight—put me on track for being a candidate for a slew of chronic illnesses. I didn't want to spend all my time going to doctor and hospital appointments, and I really didn't want to be that person who only talks about their health problems. I wanted to make big changes, and I did.

I wrote this book as a story about what happened in the year after I broke my leg. I believe stories are far more interesting and inspiring than if I wrote a book about what I think you should do to lose weight or make a change if you are over 50 and overweight. I decided to use breaking my leg as a way, metaphorically, of breaking with my past and begin to make the changes in my life that I had been longing to make a year earlier. I looked at this as an opportunity rather than something unfortunate.

This is a really positive and uplifting story filled with useful information. If you take away one thing that helps you in your quest to change your life in whatever way that might be, I will consider this little tome a huge success. I love helping and inspiring people to reach their full potential as human beings living on this planet.

Chapter Two: *Back Story*

*"Life can only be understood backwards;
but it must be lived forwards."*

—Søren Kierkegaard

How did this happen? How did I manage to gain more than 80 pounds over a 12-year period? I would ask myself these questions when I stepped onto a scale and watched the needle flutter and stop at 190 pounds. Yikes! I used to run marathons. I ran my last marathon in 1997 when I weighed 110 pounds. Even though I was a serious runner, I never made it a habit to get on a scale. I went by how my clothes fit and what size I was wearing at the time. During the mid-90s, I had completed three sub-four hour marathons—Big Sur, Boston and New York—in that order. My time for New York was 3:51, which was a pretty decent time. I was 37 when I ran my first marathon and 42 when I ran my last. I was in good shape and felt invincible. I often experienced the phenomenon known as the runner's high, and I felt like I could and would run forever. Fast-forward to 2011 and a new reality, weighing in at 190 pounds—talk about a time warp!

Again I ask, how did this happen? The 21st century started with a series of events that would form a perfect storm resulting in a massive weight gain. First, I believed that as long as I was running I could eat what I wanted and as much as I wanted. I started running less without changing my eating habits. In fact, I was such a free spirit I began to tempt fate by eating more, particularly my favorite high-calorie foods, such as bagels, ice cream and pasta. Well, my fate appeared in a gradual weight gain. I remember how my favorite pair of jeans fit a little bit tighter. This new development nagged at me, but I figured I was still running so it wouldn't matter because I would run a little farther, work a little harder. I was eating more and running less and somewhere along the line I hit 50.

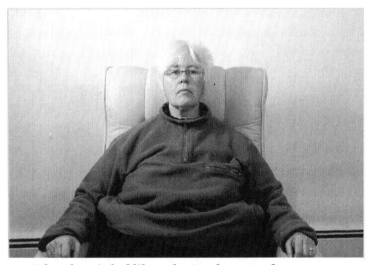

What does it feel like to be 80 plus pounds over your normal weight? The look on my face says it all.

My 50s brought an increase in my already decreasing metabolism and menopause, which just added insult to injury. Let's review: I cut back on my running, ate more, turned 50 and my metabolism was slowing down year by year. Voila! I now weighed a lot more, and that was depressing.

What does it feel like to be 80 plus pounds over your normal weight? I was tired all of the time. Naps were a welcome activity. My knees and back hurt. I felt like I moved in slow motion. I remember walking with my friend, Nancy, who, in her 80s, outpaced me. Nancy is tall, fit and walked like a speed walker. I am almost 30 years her junior, and I could not keep up with her. When I would get up from a chair I would have to use the arm rests for support to lift myself up. The sad part of the story is that although I knew I was very over-weight, I just figured I was getting older and my sore back and knees were part of the aging process. When I walked into a building I would avoid looking at my re-flection in the glass doors. I would avoid seeing old friends until I lost the weight, which never happened. I would wake up every morning and pledge to myself that today would be the day I would get my act togeth-er and start losing weight. Worst of all, I was really dis-appointed in myself, which is a sure-fire pathway to self-loathing and shame.

I was a freelance photojournalist for a large media company in New England. If you have ever watched a sporting event, or a breaking news event, you likely have seen photographers running along the sidelines trying to get their shots. This type of work is physically demanding. You might think that running with heavy gear would keep photographers in awesome physical condition. Not in my case. I managed to gain over 40 pounds during my tenure as a freelancer. Even though you are moving a lot, you are also sitting in front of a computer for hours, eating on the run and keeping odd hours. Oh, did I mention that I loved the job? I did. All I wanted to do was get the shot, and I would do pretty much anything to achieve that goal. Photojournalists all have one thing in common—get the shot, no matter what. If you are a football fan and hang around long enough after the game, you can watch the head coaches from each team looking for each other to shake hands, watch the photographers jockeying to get in position for the money shot. It is not pretty.

I remember an assignment at our local town hall. It was a selectmen's meeting, and it was located on the second floor. I climbed the two flights of stairs, and when I got to the top, I had to stop and catch my breath for 30 seconds before entering the room. I did not want to appear out of breath. I knew instinctively that I was heading down the slippery slope of deteriorating health. The state of my health could easily lead me down the path to heart disease, stroke, Type 2 diabetes or some form of cancer. I knew I had to change my lifestyle. This realization was alarming to me, yet for some reason, I could not take the necessary steps toward improving my fitness level and ultimately my health. I was like a smoker who knows smoking is bad but cannot quit, no matter how devastating the health risks.

It is an accepted fact that our metabolisms slow down as we age. According to an article put together by the ULCA nutrition professionals, Student Nutrition Awareness Campaign, "As you lose muscle mass, gain fat mass, and experience hormonal changes, your resting metabolic rate, which accounts for 65% of your daily caloric burn, will decrease. By age fifty your metabolism will be 15-20% lower than in your twenties and thirties."[1] Luckily there are things you can do to raise your metabolism to counter this decrease.

I remember being examined by my primary-care physician and asking him if there was any way to increase my metabolism; his answer was no. I am happy to report that he was wrong, because you can! This is the same doctor who wrote on my medical records that I was *morbidly obese*, yet it was never discussed or even brought up during the exam. I knew I was overweight; he knew I was overweight, but it was like the elephant in the room—it was never acknowledged. Talking to a patient about their weight is not a comfortable topic. Being overweight is directly related to the state of one's health, and I wasn't healthy. I knew the solutions to my weight problem were not going to be forthcoming from a doctor's visit. I had to initiate the process of losing weight and hold myself accountable. I could not and did not want to rely on the medical community to do it for me. I wanted to do this myself, and that is exactly what I did.

Standing at the starting line of this journey, I took a very hardcore inventory of my physical health. I am five feet and one inch tall, weighed 190 pounds and I was 55 years old at the time. Not only did I look fat, I felt old and tired. As you can imagine, I was pretty miserable about this state of affairs. I had tried several diets that not only did not work, but also backfired. I would give a diet a month or so, be unhappy with the results and find a reason to convince myself that I was happy as I was and then revert to my unhealthy eating habits. It was a vicious cycle that went on for years. We New Englanders are all about the seasons. Once April rolled around I would tell myself that I would lose 60 pounds by the first of June, just in time for summer. It never happened. I was just as overweight on June 1 as I was eight weeks earlier on April 1, and that was no joke.

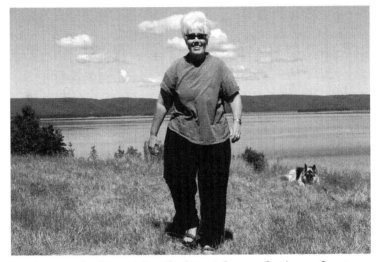

My wardrobe consisted of stretchy synthetic workout pants (one size fits all) and large T-shirts.

I didn't feel good about myself and I dressed like it. I really wanted to wear nice clothes, including a pair of fantastic fitting jeans, but when you are short and fat, nothing looks good on you. Almost all women's clothing is made of fabric that is made with some percentage of synthetic material in it. It is a sad response to the growing obesity problem in America. I once read a description of the type of pants I wore—"My life is over pants"—which means I just didn't care anymore. I did care. I just didn't have a good enough reason to change my life at the time. A good enough reason was about to appear—in a big way.

I felt hopeless about not being able to commit to losing weight. I wanted to get back to my marathon weight, but it seemed like an impossible task. I am a firm believer in that if you ask the universe to help you make a change it will respond by creating opportunities that will help you reach your goal. I asked and ignored the messages and opportunities that were presented to me. Each time you ask the messages become more powerful until you decide to make those changes. I had to have my foundation blown out from under me before I pointed myself firmly in the direction of where I wanted to go and achieve the goals I set for myself. First and foremost, I wanted to lose the 80-plus pounds that I gained over the previous 12 years. And that is exactly what I set out to do. Now, I had to make a plan and take action.

Chapter Three: *My Big Break*

"If you are going through hell, keep going."

—Winston Churchill

On the night of July 2, 2011, I was on assignment for my local newspaper in Hingham, MA. The assignment was to cover the annual Fourth of July fireworks celebration on the harbor. Hingham is a beautiful old town, located 20 miles south of Boston. As a freelance photojournalist, I have shot this event many times.

It was a beautiful warm summer night with the smell of saltwater and fried dough in the air. The sounds of patriotic music could be heard from the bandstand, together with the voices of hundreds of people singing along. The evening was charged with energy and the anticipation of the legendary fireworks display that would explode over Hingham Harbor once the night came. By the time the fireworks would start there would be thousands of spectators. People came from all over the south shore and beyond. Some arrived very early in the morning to stake out a piece of prime real estate for optimum viewing. Prior to the start of the fireworks, kids were throwing Frisbee's on the beach, people enjoyed a picnic on their blankets and boats in

29

the harbor were weighed down with folks passing the night away. It was New England at its best.

Earlier in the day I had scouted a location for my tripod. The key to shooting fireworks is to have an interesting foreground to give the photos context. Standalone shots of fireworks are pretty boring, but if you add something like boats floating in the harbor in the foreground it will be a far more interesting photograph. I had shot this assignment before and I had used boats in the harbor, so I was going for something different this time around. I had stopped by a house located high up on a hill overlooking the harbor, and I knew it would have a much different perspective and foreground than previous years. I asked the owner of the property for permission to shoot from there later in the evening and he generously said yes. Shooting fireworks requires a lot of preparation, especially if you are looking to get the money shot. My plan was to set up my tripod around 8:45 p.m., allowing me to have my camera ready to go. Before the fireworks I had to get some celebration shots of people having fun and celebrating the Fourth on the beach.

I made my way through the crowd looking for fun shots. The possibilities were endless. They included people wearing Fourth of July hats, T-shirts or waving flags along to the beat of the music. There also were folks eating giant pieces of fried dough covered in powdered sugar, kids having their faces painted, or like my neighbors, John and Janet, playing a game of backgammon on their beach blanket. A group of teens begged me to take their picture, and I took a few frames of them jumping in the air and acting crazy. They loved it. I followed the shoreline all the while taking photos of kids searching for starfish and sand dollars. The tide was dead low and I soon found myself standing in front of the seawall. The entire face of the 15-foot seawall was exposed. I was looking for shots when I spotted three girls sitting on top of the seawall and eating ice cream. The sun was beginning to fade and cast a pink and orange light, making this a perfect photo op. I was shooting with my Nikon D3 camera along with a 70-200 mm lens. Together, these two pieces of gear weighed almost six pounds, and until this night they were my priority, meaning I protected them more than anything, including myself.

I took a few frames of the girls eating ice cream on the seawall. They were oblivious of me. I looked at my LCD screen and knew I could do better if I moved farther to the left allowing for a better angle and revealing more of their faces. What happened next would propel me on a journey that I had never imagined.

As I stepped to my left, I did not realize that my right foot had settled in the low tide mud, creating a suction effect. As I turned to my left, my right foot stayed while I held my camera with my left hand, causing me to lose my balance. As I began to fall, I was trying to prevent my camera from landing in the mud. This would prove to be unfortunate, because as I fell, I felt three very quick snaps in my right leg in what seemed like a fraction of a second. They say when you break a bone you know it right away, and I did. I also knew it was a terrible break because my right foot was pointing away from me in a direction that was not in my normal range of motion. My right foot had essentially detached from my right leg. I was in shock.

As I lay on the beach, my right hand covering my injured leg for protection, I called out for help. Although there were thousands of people attending the event, there was no one around me. I kept calling out for help for what seemed an eternity. I kept saying to anyone within earshot, "I need help; I have broken my leg," over and over again to no avail. People saw me lying on the beach, but they did not think I was seriously hurt. My friend, Suzanne, who is a psychologist, told me about "Bystander's Syndrome." When people attend an event or go someplace for a specific reason, they tend to focus on the actual event to the exclusion of all else. In my case, people were there to celebrate the Fourth of July, not to see or hear me lying on the beach calling out for help.

Finally, a man came over to help me. I was still in shock, and although I was visibly upset, I wasn't crying, because the pain hadn't yet begun to register. I felt like I had met this man before. As it turned out he was a first responder from Pembroke, a nearby town where I had shot many assignments. He kept me calm until the Hingham Fire Department emergency medical technicians arrived. Everything happened quickly after their arrival. They strapped me onto a hard board and then onto a gurney. Several, self-described handsome firemen (they were) carried me up off the beach and put me into an ambulance for the ride to nearby South Shore Hospital in Weymouth, the next town over from

Hingham. As we were riding to the hospital the pain in my leg was beginning to make itself known in a big way. The EMT asked me if I wanted something for the pain. Yes, please! Once he located a vein in my arm, he gave me a shot of something to take the edge off until we arrived at the hospital. In recent years, I had been told that I have small veins because they were always hard to find. As it turns out, I have normal- size veins that were located under a very thick layer of fat. I didn't know it at the time, but I was creating a mental list of reasons why I should lose weight. They remained in my subconscious until I began my recovery in the coming months.

While riding to the hospital in the back of the ambulance I called my partner, Linda, to let her know that I had broken my leg. When I think about it now I can't believe I had the wherewithal to make the call. It is just another example of technology and the world we live in today. Of course, our technological world is far from perfect, especially after I got a dropped call in mid-conversation! I was able to say that I broke my leg and then nothing. The EMT said calls always dropped out in that area and to try again when we passed through Jackson Square in Weymouth. Sure enough, I got through and let Linda know what had happened and where I was headed.

As I lay on a gurney near the nurse's station in the emergency room of South Shore Hospital, my leg was beginning to throb. Linda arrived wearing an expression of horror, sorrow and worry on her face. She quickly scooped up my camera gear and spoke to the nurse regarding my state. The nurse realized I was in need of something for my pain and proceeded to give me my first injection of Dilaudid, a very powerful painkiller. I remember the drug traveled first to my brain and then to my leg—ah, instant relief. Although the pain disappeared, the side effect was intense nausea that hit me like an oncoming train. And that train stayed with me for the next four days.

Next up were X-rays. I remember that I was wheeled down a long corridor and parked outside a nondescript door. I felt like I was in a scene right out of a Robin Cook novel. There was no one around and the fluorescent lights only added to the creepiness. Meanwhile, I continued to retch my brains out while waiting to be X-rayed. Soon the door opened and the nighttime X-ray technician came out and wheeled me into the room. I knew she wasn't too happy with me because I was so sick. Oh well, it is a hospital after all, and it wasn't exactly fun for me either.

Following the X-rays I soon found myself in a small room with a doctor, nurse and Linda. The doctor, who was very kind, explained that he was going to set my leg. Fortunately, I was so out of it that all I remember is the doctor holding my right leg up by my big toe and wiggling my foot and leg into place. I am told the pain would have been excruciating had I not been medicated. Thankfully, I was blissfully drugged out because I don't remember feeling any pain.

After setting my leg, the South Shore staff decided to send me to another hospital. It was the Fourth of July weekend and my leg injury was so severe that there was no one available locally to handle my case. I rode in an ambulance to Brigham and Women's Hospital in Boston, a world-class hospital with a world-class orthopedic trauma team. This was a perfect example of divine intervention because I was so out of it that decisions were being made without my input. I just let it go, and after a bumpy ride to Boston I found myself in the very capable hands of the staff at the Brigham, as it is known locally. If you are seriously injured this is where you want to be treated.

The orthopedic trauma team was impressed with how the medical team at South Shore Hospital had set my leg but not enough to not reset it after another round of X-rays in an eerily similar fluorescent-lit corridor. It was the wee hours of the next morning and the lone X-ray tech came out to roll me in for round two.

The last thing I remember was someone cutting my clothes off of me. It is funny the things that go through your mind. I was thinking that I was glad I had showered, shaved my legs and had freshly painted toes before descending into darkness. The next next stop was my hospital room, my home for the next six days.

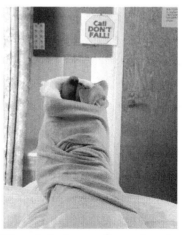

My painted toenails peek out from the cast.

Once I woke up and realized that I could not get out of my hospital bed, reality began to set in. If you cannot get up that means no restroom and that means the dreaded bedpan. Having someone shove a bedpan under my butt was sobering and humiliating. I made another mental note to add this experience to my list of reasons to lose weight. For part of my stay I had a roommate whose idea of a vacation was a week's stint in the hospital. She had the television on 24/7. Normally this would have driven me crazy, but I was so medicated that I didn't care. This person was so disruptive that a nurse came in the middle of the night. She was holding a book. She pulled a piece of paper out of the book and held it up for me to read. The paper read, "Would you like to move to another room?" I declined; at that point I didn't care. I did later.

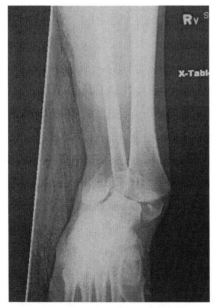

X-ray showing the broken bones.

The health-team at Brigham and Women's is the best. I knew this based on my own experience, but a medical technician who was temping at the hospital confirmed it. "The nurses are really great," he said. "I know because I work at a lot of hospitals and there are some nasty nurses out there." Every member of the health team—nurses, doctors, technicians and maintenance folks—could not have been more professional and kind.

The doctors decided the swelling in my leg had subsided enough to schedule surgery on July 4th. While I was lying in bed digesting this development, I decided to get my iPhone out and open my Facebook app. I do not normally share very personal information but I decided to update my status with the following statement.

"Okay, Facebook friends, I am sharing my latest photography adventure. Slipped and broke my leg in three places at the Hingham Fourth of July Celebration last night. I normally don't share this type of info, but I am having surgery tomorrow and could use some healing energy sent my way. I am at Brigham and Women's Hospital and they are great. Thanks in advance!"

I received a lot of kind words and positive energy sent my way. My friend, Jeff Bossio, sent the following:

"Your toes do look nasty. I had surgery on my ankle 4 broken places - You'll B great. And in no time running and taking pics again. How u feel is dictated by the way u think. Sending positive energy, embrace it be strong and optimistic."

I would take this message from Jeff and run with it. I made the decision to look at this injury as a great and positive experience. By making this decision, I paved the long road to recovery in the most optimistic and affirming terms. I embraced my injury and was strong and hopeful.

A few days after my surgery, Jason, a physical thera-pist, showed up in my room with a set of crutches and an air boot. It was time to get out of bed for the first time. Also, I was able to use the restroom! Yahoo! Yes, I know it is the little things in life that make us happy. However, this was huge for me at the time. It also meant I was one step closer to getting out of the hospital and on the road to recovery. First, I had to pass a test before they would release me. It is a kind of gradu-ation ceremony. I had to put on an extra Johnny to cover my very ample butt. Yes, you guessed it; another reason was added to the growing list of reasons to lose weight. Jason and I made our way down two very long corridors to where the wooden staircase was located. The staircase had only three steps, but it may as well have been the stairway to the Empire State Building. In order to pass the test, I had to scale these steps using my crutches and then come back down. Sounds simple, right? Not really! The steps seemed like they were 50 feet tall and I was five feet tall, which I am. Balancing my very overweight body on two little rubber nubs while climbing these steps scared the hell out of me.

I passed the test, graduated and was on my way home to begin my recovery.

Chapter Four: *Decision Time*

"Change your thoughts and you change your world." — Norman Vincent Peale

Once I came home from the hospital reality set in. What I mean by this is that I would be spending my summer either sitting on my butt or lying on my back. The doctor's instructions were very clear: "You cannot put any weight on your right leg for three months." Unlike a single clean break where your leg is wrapped in a cast for everyone to sign, I was given an air boot that I could remove when I was not moving around. This is because the eleven pins and two plates inserted into my right leg and ankle required two incisions, one on each side of my ankle. You can't have two incisions with stitches in your leg wrapped in plaster. Therefore, the healing process takes much longer. My leg could not support me until all three breaks had healed. That being said, I am very glad that I live in the 21st century where medicine has developed to the point where having a lot of hardware in my leg and ankle would enable me to walk normally again.

My exercise would be using my walker to hobble from one room to the other, making sure I didn't put weight on my injured leg. I lived in a one-floor apartment, so my workout was going to be minimal at best. One footnote (pun intended) was that my apartment was originally designed for an elderly person. It was small, one level with two steps leading to the front door. The bathroom had wall bars and a shower that could easily fit a folding chair on the inside. These are the things that take on a larger-than-life quality when life throws you a curveball. I would be sitting down for all of my showers for the next four months.

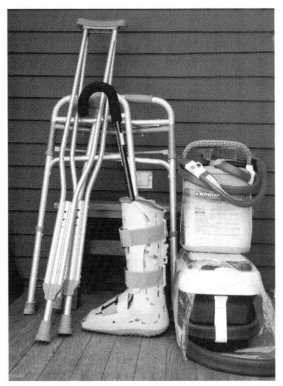

These items became very important to me in the next several months. They allowed me some semblance of mobility, be it very slow.

The two steps leading up to my front door would make my life exponentially easier, but initially they seemed insurmountable. The perspective from moving around on crutches changes everything, from depth perception, balance, and of course, fear of falling. The first time I arrived home from the hospital, I literally sat down on the first step and moved backward up to the second. It was the first of many awkward and humbling experiences. It would take me a while to get used to moving around on a walker and crutches. It is not as easy as it looks. Also carrying an extra 80 pounds around definitely added to the effort of transporting myself from one place to another.

Knowing that I would be spending the summer not expending much energy, I made a decision to eliminate food products made with refined sugar or corn syrup. Usually, when people come to visit they want to bring food, especially baked goods. I will state here that I am unequivocally a sugar addict. I love candy, desserts of any kind, and generally all things sweet and delicious. I knew if I did not give up these delectable delights I would easily gain 20 pounds or more during my three-month layoff. I could not afford to do this because I was already 80 pounds overweight, and according to my primary care physician, *"morbidly obese."* Once I made the decision to give up cakes, cookies, candy and ice cream, I put out the word to folks coming to visit: "I gratefully ask that you please not bring treats." Everyone was great about this and they helpfully complied. I lost eight pounds sitting on my ass all summer, thanks to my making a clear and decisive decision to eliminate refined sugar from my diet. It would be a decision that I would hold onto even now.

The first decision I made prior to giving up sugar was the one that would pave the way to a beautiful and successful recovery. I decided to look at breaking my leg as a truly positive experience, an opportunity to make a powerful and meaningful change in my life. Or as the animated character, Homer Simpson would say, "This is a crisitunity," a point where a crisis meets an opportunity. I was in crisis and the potential for opportunity was unlimited and up to me. I was not going to complain or feel sorry for myself. There would be no pity party for me. This is one of the best decisions I have ever made. It was practical and instructive. Also, by staying positive and upbeat meant I could handle any and all adversity that came my way—with ease. This was not in any way a trip down the river of denial or an impersonation of Pollyanna. No way! Breaking my leg meant three months of sitting or lying down, inability to work, four months of physical therapy and a whole lot of pain. I wasn't denying reality by being upbeat and positive. I was using being positive as a tool for helping me through what could have been a very dark period of my life and what actually turned out to be the best thing that ever happened to me.

I will be referring to the tools I used to help me through this experience as my personal toolbox. The tools I used are personal to me but can be used by anyone. So far the tools that I have in my personal toolbox are *decisiveness* and *the power of positive thinking*. I might even refer to them as *power tools* because of how effective they were for me.

Another fantastic tool that holds a prominent place in my toolbox is the *thought renewal* tool. Thought renewal is when you change the way you think and speak, from negative to positive. This sounds so simple, and it is, but it is also challenging. It is in our nature to be judgmental, to be critical of others and generally complain about things. I am guilty of all three, so you know that I am challenged (in oh so many ways).

There is a method to thought renewal that works. Step one: I have decided to look at my injury and recovery experience in a positive way, which means I am going to speak in those terms. Example: A friend comes for a visit and they ask me how I am doing. I respond in the following manner, I say, "I am in tremendous pain, I can't work, I can't walk, I can't drive, why did this happen to me?" Insert tears and music here for effect. As you can imagine, my visitor is wondering how she can come up with a good excuse to make a quick exit, because this visit is downright depressing. *"I want out of here and I am not coming back!"* Now reverse the situation, and my visitor asks me the same question, "How are you doing?" My response is completely different. I say, "I am great! I am so fortunate that I will be able to walk again. I live in a perfect place for healing, and I am so lucky to have friends and family to care for and visit with me. I am realizing that breaking my leg is probably the best thing that ever happened to me because it is an opportunity to make some positive changes in my life, changes that have been a long time coming. Life is good!" My visitor's response is, *"Wow, hallelujah, I must be at a revival meeting because this person is taking this experience really well, and I am feeling better about my life, too! I want to hang out with Laura because her positive attitude is rubbing off on me!"*

I had many of these types of visits over the course of the summer. It was one of those totally unexpected silver linings to being out of commission for three months. I call them my long, lazy summer afternoon conversations with friends and family. In today's fast-paced world with emails, texts, phone calls and tweets, there is no substitute for a good old-fashioned, face-to-face visit with deep and meaningful conversation. These visits were refreshing and luxurious. Some of these visits lasted for hours. I had face time with friends I hadn't seen in years. The world slowed down even for just an afternoon. Some of my visits would last from when the sun was high in the sky to a slow room-darkening sunset. Spectacular!

Chapter Five: *Turning Back The Clock*

> *"Time is a very healing place,*
> *one in which you can grow."*
>
> —Denise Tanner

As I mentioned, I somehow managed to gain more than 80 pounds over a 12-year period. I am a veteran marathon runner who completed three major marathons, Big Sur, Boston and New York. I ran my last marathon in 1997, and let's just say *that was then and this is now.*

During the spring before my accident, I decided to change primary-care physicians and part of the process was picking up my medical records to bring with me to my new doctor. I read through the pile of documents and came to the part where I was listed as *morbidly obese.* The term, morbidly obese, refers to people who are 50% -100% over their normal body weight. Whoa! I knew I was overweight, but it never occurred to me that I was *morbidly obese* because I didn't go near a scale for years. Reading those words was unnerving and depressing. Switching doctors happened a few months prior to my accident, and although intellectually, I was aware of my *morbidly obese* status, I still was unable to get my butt in gear to do anything about it.

When I ran my last marathon in 1997, I weighed 110 pounds. In 2011, I weighed 190 pounds. I find it therapeutic to share these numbers. There is such a premium put on how much we weigh, and there are so many forces that constantly compete against being at an optimum weight. People who are overweight are embarrassed and ashamed about how they look and feel, and I was one of those people. Being able to admit to myself that I weighed 190 pounds was a relief and a solid reason to take the first steps to change this state of mind. I know I am part of the majority because everyone I know or come in contact with is dissatisfied with how much they weigh and how they look. This pertains to thin people as well as overweight people. Society has set the parameters for what looks good and we go right along. Rubenesque is not in vogue these days. There is one thing we all have in common—we all want to be thin!

Growing up in my house, every celebration, holiday, funeral, you name it, revolved around food. My mother was a fabulous cook. Not only my mother, but also my father and two brothers all liked to cook and bake. I was the only one who did not, and to this day I still do not like to cook. I do like to eat, though. Who doesn't? In my formative years food became a very important part of my life. It was my drug of choice, one that I turned to for comfort and solace.

Fast forward to July 2, 2011, and I am at a crossroads. I had already made the decision to give up products made with refined sugar and corn syrup. The only sugar I was going to eat would be in fruit. Unbeknownst to me, this was the unofficial beginning of my journey to lose the weight and turn back the clock to when I was a healthy person who ran marathons. Also, I did not realize (ignorance is bliss) that it would take more than a year of patience, hard work and discipline to lose the weight that I had gained over 12 years. Opportunity had knocked, and I could choose to continue along the path of my life as a *morbidly obese* person or I could use breaking my leg as a metaphor and break with this way of life, make a major change in my life and redirect how I wanted to live it. Which path would I take? I chose the latter. I decided to change my relationship with food and make the commitment to lose the weight and get super fit in the process.

Initially, giving up sugar was made easier by the fact that I was captive for three months, unable to do more than move in small circles around my apartment, using my trusty walker. I couldn't drive, work, walk or do much of anything on my own. My edict of no one bringing desserts into the house also helped. There were a few times when I wanted to have some ice cream because it was summer and ice cream always tastes better in the hot weather. These cravings didn't rear themselves until the middle of August, and by then I was already six weeks in. I knew if I caved I would be super disappointed in myself. So I didn't cave. The cravings eventually passed along with the rest of the summer.

Two weeks after I was home from the hospital, my partner Linda and I went out to dinner. It was my virgin trip out into the real world on my crutches. Up until this point I was just using my walker, but crutches are much easier for travel. My brother, Joe, helped me out the door and over to the car—no small feat. I backed myself into the back seat of the car. This sounds so simple, but here I am, all of my bulk, teetering on the two tiny rubber nubs on my crutches. This was frightening because of the balance issue. I was given strict instructions not to put weight on my right leg, and if I touched down I could further damage my injured leg, which could cause all sorts of problems and prolong my recovery. The simple act of going out to my car and getting in it became this big deal. The point here is that I took for granted my ability and agility for completing even the most mundane tasks. I now had to think about things my brain usually did on autopilot. Carrying an extra 80 pounds around on crutches made matters much more difficult. This was another reason to add to the growing list of reasons to lose the weight. The list was getting longer every day.

We arrived to the restaurant and Linda let me off near the front door. I made my way up the walkway and found myself confronting the reality of a handicapped person in a public space. The door to the restaurant opened out, and I was unable to balance my crutches while pulling the door open. Luckily, a stranger leaving the building held the door open for me. I found a place in the foyer where I could sit and wait. As I waited, I thought about how challenging it is for those who are permanently handicapped. It is sobering, and I now know that the term "handicapped access" has many meanings—and not always what you expect.

We were seated at a table on the other side of the bar. The waitress came over with a bottle of wine under her arm. They were having a wine promotion and she asked us if we would like to participate. I pointed to my crutches and told her it wouldn't be pretty if I had a few glasses of wine. I knew that drinking was off limits until I was off the meds and the crutches. I am not much of a drinker, and besides alcohol usually leads to poor food choices.

As I looked over the menu there was a picture of a steak and mashed potatoes on the cover. All of a sudden I had a mad craving for beef. I did not order the steak, but the cravings for meat did not go away, they only intensified. This was really weird for me because I rarely ate meat, except for the occasional burger. Now I had a craving for red meat and mashed potatoes, and it wasn't going away. Over the next six weeks, I had steak tips and mashed potatoes six times at six different restaurants. We ate a lot of takeout because Linda was super busy with her work, and she had to take care of me before she left for work and when she came home. It became a contest of which establishment had the best steak tips and mashed potatoes. The winner hands down was Jamie's Pub in North Scituate, Massachusetts! Toward the end of September, the meat cravings disappeared. I believe that the cravings were the result of my changing diet and reduction in sugar intake. The steak and potatoes also served as comfort food.

The only limitation to my diet was that I was no longer going to eat products made with refined sugar and corn syrup. Everything else was up for grabs. I ate a healthy diet of fruits, salads, good carbs and pizza once a week. In retrospect, this was the foundation for a new way of eating and changing my relationship with food. I would take the long view as well as change what I ate very slowly over a long period of time of a year or more. This is one of the major tools for my success in losing weight and keeping it off. I didn't want to be on a "diet." I wanted to develop a new way of eating that would basically stay the same even after I reached my goal. I refer to this as *sustainable eating*.

As July led into August, my mindset was one of patience and focus. I was experiencing tremendous pain in my leg, but I knew that each day that passed brought me one step closer to October 4, the day I would finally put weight on my right leg. Yeah!

I remember going to my first follow-up appointment with Dr. Michael Weaver at Brigham and Women's Hospital two weeks after my surgery. I would have the stitches removed from the two incisions in my leg following an X-ray. When I saw the X-ray of my leg that showed the eleven pins and two plates, I was shocked. My ankle looked like the bionic man. It was at this point that the gravity of my injury really hit home and that my life was changing at a fast and furious pace.

Before my appointment I met a woman who was at the hospital for her six-week appointment. She had been cleaning the windows on the side of her RV while standing on a ladder. As she came down she missed the last step and broke her leg in several places. I remember being envious of her because she was four weeks ahead of me in the recovery department. I kept telling myself, *"patience and focus, patience and focus."*

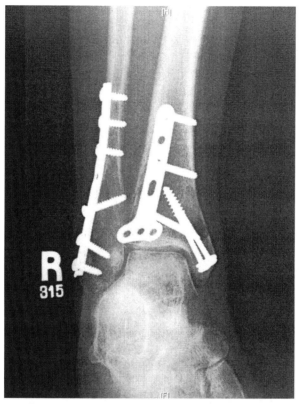

The X-ray of my leg showed the eleven pins and two plates. What a shock! I felt extremely lucky to be living in the 21st century.

My eating habits continued to improve as time went on. The longer I went without sugar the less I craved it. It also helped that Linda prepared good healthy food for me. My relationship with food was changing, and I was still taking baby steps. The only real plan at this point was the elimination of sugary junk food until I got the go ahead to work out, and this wouldn't be happening for another few months, on November 1. In the meantime, I focused on not putting weight on my right leg. I fell a couple of times trying not to. I would tell myself, *"I'm okay, I'm okay."* A friend once asked me if during those three months, didn't I try to put weight on my right leg just to see how it would feel. Absolutely not! Fear is a good motivator and I wanted to walk again like a normal person.

As October 4 neared I was getting anxious to get on with my life. I figured once I could put weight on my leg, I would be off and running. This was not to be. I did take the first few steps with my physical therapist by my side that fall morning, and to say it was anticlimactic would be an understatement. There was a searing pain followed by the realization that it was going to take a lot longer to even walk with crutches. Instead, it would be two crutches, one crutch, a cane and then several more months learning how to walk again. I knew I could handle all that was happening, but I never dreamed my biggest challenge was going to be learning how to walk again. Before the accident I walked my whole life without ever thinking about it. We take this movement for granted, but when you break down the mechanics of how we walk and then really think about it, it is a total challenge! I am lucky, because with a lot of hard work I knew I would be able to walk again, especially with my terrific and talented physical therapists, Susan and Terrence, by my side. Physical therapists fall into the unsung hero's category in my book. Without them I would not be where I am today. This experience gave me greater understanding, respect and boundless empathy for those people who have permanent disabilities.

On October 30, Dr. Weaver told me the bones were healed and that I could go to the gym unrestricted—nothing was off-limits. Now the real work began. I had joined a small gym the previous February and my membership was still valid. Like many folks who join a gym in January or February, I went for a month and never went back. I didn't like it, so I quit. Fast forward to October 30, and I wanted to get back to the gym in the worst way. I have a new saying, "If you can't, you want," and I wanted with the attitude and enthusiasm of a person who just received a new lease on life. I was now on my way to evolving from a person who was *morbidly obese* to one who is super fit.

Chapter Six:
Counting, Measuring & Recording

**"As you grow older, make sure you count two
things, your calories and your blessings."**

—Unknown

I will now answer the question I am asked most.
"How did you do it? How did you lose all that
weight?" I can't tell you how many people—friends,
family, complete strangers—come up to me and ask
these questions.

When I was given the go ahead to work out unrestricted at the gym, I was elated. My bones had healed, but I
had zero muscle strength in my right leg. All the muscle tissue had atrophied during the three months I was
sitting around my house. The saying, "Use it or lose it,"
certainly applied in this situation. The muscle tissue in
my leg disappeared, and I had no stamina. I literally
didn't have a leg to stand on because there was no
muscle in my leg to support my body, which meant I
still had to use crutches to get around—time for a new
plan.

I arrived at my gym on crutches, which drew a look of
consternation from the person at the front desk. I think
they were worried I might fall over and hurt myself—

again. Little did they know that I had morphed into one of the most fearful and careful people on the planet. My first day at the gym, I managed to do seven minutes on the recumbent bicycle. Yeah! When I say I started from the beginning, I wasn't kidding.

Numbers Game

I ran into my friend, Lori, one day as I was coming home from the gym. I told her about my goals, particularly my weight-loss goal. She suggested Weight Watchers because she had experienced success with this program. You could either sign up at a local bricks-and-mortar storefront or register for their online program. I went home and did a bit of research online about Weight Watchers. As I was surfing the Internet, I came across a blog that not only reviewed Weight Watchers but also a few other weight-loss programs. One of those programs was My Fitness Pal, a calorie counter and diet-tracking site. The blogger gave Weight Watchers high marks but was also impressed with My Fitness Pal because it, too, was an excellent program with one key difference—it was free! This was the deal breaker for me because I couldn't work; therefore, finances were an issue. I signed on. There are many online calorie counting programs to choose from such as Lose It, SparkPeople Calorie Counter, The Daily Plate, iGoogle Calorie Counter, and Calorie Count to name a few. I chose My Fitness Pal because it was not only free but it appeared in front of me at the right time. All of these websites share two common threads. Their software enables you to count food calories and burned calories through exercise and a community of like-minded individuals to share experiences and advice.

I consider the incorporation of My Fitness Pal into my weight loss plan to be the most important component to my success. The numbers don't lie. Once I set up an account with a username and password I got to work. I added my then current height and weight and my goal weight. The program takes your numbers and calculates how many calories you would need each day to lose the weight. Each day I would enter everything I ate and how much. The program would automatically calculate this information into calories. There is a database of every food imaginable, and if it isn't there, you can add a food. Members are constantly adding and updating to the database. My Fitness Pal is the equivalent of a good old-fashioned food journal, except it's easier and more gratifying! Instead of writing by hand in a notebook and trying to figure out the number of calories you have eaten, they do it for you. This alone makes the success ratio go up exponentially.

Another great tool that the program offers is the ability to add in the calories that you burn from your workouts to that of your daily allotment. This was key to my success at losing weight over an extended period of time. For example, my daily calorie allotment was 1330 calories, add onto this number 550 calories from my workout on The Arc Trainer and now you are at 1880 calories. I rarely ate back my exercise calories while I was in the losing phase, and when I did, it was only a portion. I believe this accelerated my weight loss.

Almost all online calorie counting websites are designed as social media sites, My Fitness Pal included. You can add friends, troll the message boards, update your status and make comments about your friend's updates. During the first few months I would keep track of my food intake and mainly look in on the "Success Stories" category in the community. I loved this place because the members would post their before and after photos along with a few lines about how they lost their weight. Other members would post positive and supportive comments. I found this to be informative, helpful and inspirational. There were comments from members of all ages and from all over the world. It is a safe place for people to express themselves while they work toward their goal of losing weight. Using an online food journal like My Fitness Pal is a very important tool in my toolbox. It keeps me honest about what I am eating and gives me a visual accounting of my progress 365 days of the year.

One of the biggest eye openers for me was learning just how many calories are in the foods I eat and used to eat. For instance, one of my favorite foods is a sesame bagel. There are 350 calories in a sesame bagel, and that is with nothing on it! Also, there is no nutritional value in a sesame bagel. I used to eat a whole bagel with a lot of peanut butter on it. By the way, one tablespoon of peanut butter has 95 calories in it. I probably slathered 3-4 tablespoons on my bagel, which would bring that bagel calorie count up to somewhere around 650-750. This would account for half my allotted calories for the day! Now, I rarely eat bagels, and I measure out any peanut butter that I eat. Measuring and weighing food as well as being mindful of portion control are half the battle toward losing weight. I would even state that it is more than half the battle.

I decided to change my relationship with food because if I did not, I would land right back where I started— *morbidly obese*. As I mentioned earlier, in my house growing up, food was central to every event or celebration. Thanksgiving was my mother's time to shine and shine she did. She cooked enough food to feed an army, except there were usually just eight to ten people seated around the dinner table. My mother would not only cook a complete turkey dinner with all the fixings, but she also wanted our heritage to be represented with a full menu of Italian fare. This included pasta, eggplant with Parmesan and braciola. This was just the main entree. Before we hit the dining room, we all sat around the living room coffee table that groaned under the weight of the fruit and nut bowl, potato chips with onion dip, my mother's homemade fudge and an assortment of other delectable delights. Following dinner, the array of desserts was irresistible, but by then we were all sprawled out on the couch in a food coma. It must have been the tryptophan in the turkey that made us tired—um, no. We just ate too much. The calorie count for those Thanksgiving's was off the charts, unimaginable.

To reach my weight loss goal and become super fit I had to not only change my relationship with food but also make a sea change in my eating habits. I began eliminating most of the junk food from my diet over a long period of time. It wasn't all or nothing. This never worked for me before. I still eat pizza, the occasional burger and dessert. The difference is that I budget my daily caloric intake to accommodate the increase in calories that these foods literally bring to the table. I do not read articles about food or restaurant reviews or watch cooking shows. The power of suggestion has a great influence on my mind. This is why marketing is so effective. If I watch a cooking show and they are making something that sounds delicious, there is no doubt in my mind that I want it. I ask myself, is it worth watching this show and tempting fate? The answer is no. We are bombarded with marketing and advertising messages every day from so many sources that half the time we are not even aware of it. I have chosen to become aware when it comes to food. We keep only healthy food in the house. The reality is that even when you are in the zone of losing weight and you feel great, having foods around that tempt you only serves as a reminder that this is a lifetime change and that you could go over to the other side in a heartbeat. It is a sad but true fact.

I remember listening to a Tony Robbins motivation program many years ago and he threw out a challenge to his listeners. The next time you go to a party or an event, do not eat or drink anything except a glass of water. Sound Draconian? I don't think so. It is only food. I try to do this more often than not. Sometimes I will have a glass of wine or beer. The food at these events is usually high in calorie and not worth the guilt you will feel the next day.

A thread started on one of the My Fitness Pal message boards went like this, "How are you going to celebrate when you reach your goal?" A lot of people said they would celebrate with eating some of their favorite foods (translation: high in calories). I thought this was interesting and asked myself the same question. I answered; I would buy some new clothes, particularly a great pair of jeans. If I celebrated with food it would not square up with my goal of changing my relationship with food. I worked hard to lose weight, and I want to make it a permanent change, so I chose a non-food way to celebrate. I bought two pairs of size 6 skinny jeans at Old Navy. I felt like I was living in a different universe that October day.

There is no mystery to losing weight. It is calories in versus calories out. The folks who design calorie-counting websites encourage participants to lose weight at a reasonable pace and also to look at it as a lifestyle change rather than a quick-fix diet. We all know quick-fix diets almost never work. I know this firsthand, because I have struggled with my weight almost my entire life.

Only fifteen percent of Americans know how many calories they should consume each day. This accounts for the obesity problem in this country. I had no idea how many calories I should eat each day, and I also did not know how many calories I was eating each day. Ignorance is bliss until you become *morbidly obese*, and then not so much. I weigh the foods I eat. I count how many glasses of water I drink per day. I log everything I put into my mouth into my account with My Fitness

Pal. My last entry is at night when I complete my totals for the day and I am under, or at, my calorie allotment. This is a very important tool that I use for managing and maintaining my weight. It may seem like a lot of work, but it isn't. It only takes a few minutes of my day. I love it because I am in total control and it keeps me honest. Counting calories is a form of personal empowerment. I consider counting calories to be one of the most important tools for losing weight.

Chapter Seven: *A Nation of Addicts*

"Every form of addiction is bad,
no matter whether the narcotic be alcohol,
morphine or idealism." –C.G. Jung

One of the dirty little secrets of our time is that we are addicted to sugar, salt and fat. There is a lot written about this but not nearly enough attention has been drawn to the fact that the food industry spends billions of dollars trying to make Americans and people all over the world addicted to their food products. Giant food corporations hire scientists, psychologists and chemists to figure out just how to create products that lure the average individual into not only purchasing their products but also becoming addicted to them. This is their business and they are doing nothing illegal. I am not going to go into detail about how the mad scientists operate behind the food industry-curtain. I will talk about how we are a nation of food addicts and until we understand our addictions we will never be able to successfully lose weight.

I have already said I am addicted to sugar. It has been reported that sugar is as addictive as cocaine, heroin or alcohol. This is no joke or an overly dramatic statement. The food industry mantra is, "When in doubt add sugar." And boy, do they ever. Sugar, salt and fat are the darlings of the pleasure centers of your brain. Once your brain gets a taste for one or all three of these items you want more and you want it now. Fruit juice is loaded with sugar and not the natural kind you might think. Every time a mother gives her child a juice box or a bottle of apple juice she may not be aware that there are oftentimes more than 12 teaspoons of sugar in each bottle. This is not exactly the healthy juice product you believed it to be. Children are targeted early and often. Once they have a sugary product they want it again and again, well into adulthood.

If you want to lose weight and keep it off you have to take a hard look at the foods you love to eat and figure out if you are addicted to them. Once you establish this fact then you can either do something about it or not. I can attest that it is not easy to live with my sugar addiction. My goal is to eat clean 90 percent of the time and allow for a treat day every two weeks. My treat involves ice cream, cupcakes or both. I look forward to these treats like an addict looking for her next fix—sad but true. I am being brutally honest here. My brain talks to me about sugar. When this happens I think of the movie, *A Beautiful Mind*, starring Russell Crowe. Crowe's character was haunted by delusions of people he thought were following him, but in reality they were figments of his imagination. Wherever he went they went with him. It wasn't until the end of the movie that he made peace with these imaginary people. In the film they are shown off to the side, just hanging out. The point is they were still there, but he accepted their existence and learned to live with them. I use this analogy for my sugar addiction. I have made peace with it and it is still there and probably always will be as long as I live. I am still learning how to live with sugar addiction. I do not diminish the tragedy of any type of addiction, but being addicted to sugar has been scientifically proven to have a negative effect on the mind and body.

I was visiting a client for a photography project I was working on. She had mentioned that I somehow looked different. I hadn't seen her in over a year, and when I did, I was down 30 pounds in my weight loss journey. While at the office one of her colleagues came in holding two slices of steaming hot pizza. The aroma was intoxicating. When he left she told me that the new management in their company cafeteria served this new pizza. She then proceeded to ask me how I was losing the weight and what I ate. Our meeting came to a close and she walked me to the elevator, which was located across from the cafeteria. She told me she was going to get some of that delicious pizza for her lunch. This was after her telling me how much she wanted to lose weight! That pizza was like a siren calling her name, and she couldn't resist. I understand this scenario completely. This is what we are up against—the sights, smells and sounds of every cafeteria, food establishment and supermarket luring us into their web of food, or what is referred to as food. It can be overwhelming, but there are tools to help us avoid going down the path of no resistance.

The first step is not to have your favorite foods in the house. If you want them, you have to go get them. If you live in New England like I do and the weather is cold and miserable a lot of the year, chances are you won't go out and procure that candy, ice cream or salty snack. Get your family on board. Without the support of family, the rate of success plummets. If they want the types of foods you are trying to avoid and they end up on your shopping list, you have just set yourself up for failure. This is why I advocate baby steps and the process of elimination. This is not an all-or-nothing process. It has to be slow and steady. I gave up sugary desserts during my three months of recovery, but I ate whatever else I wanted. Once I got on my feet, literally, I began to eliminate processed foods that nine times out of ten included sugar and corn syrup in the ingredients. As my weight continued to go down, my desire to eat clean, healthier foods went up. I eat food that for the most part has one ingredient. I am not a purist, but I strive to eat for good health, in moderation and to get the biggest bang for my buck, energy wise. It requires the management skills that are used to run a successful business. My business these days is to keep the weight off, have optimum energy and to be super fit.

I changed my relationship with food. This is an on-going process and challenge. If I didn't change my relationship with food and break some of my life long habits, I would not have been successful in my weight loss. I am a New England Patriots football fan, and in the fall when game time rolled around, the immediate thought was, "What do we want to eat during the game?" Sports and television go hand in hand with eating all kinds of high-calorie junk food. Things like chicken wings, chips and salsa, pizza—you name it! Drinking beer also is high on the list. I find that after a few beers any rational thought goes out the window and bad food choices loom on the horizon. The calorie count went through the roof and suddenly I just added a few extra pounds onto an already overburdened body. Something had to change. I needed to break this habit.

Instead of eating junk food and drinking beer, I changed direction. I would eat a good meal during the game instead of mindlessly munching on whatever delectable salty snack or sweet treat was in front of me. Sometimes I didn't eat or drink anything—what a concept! It may not seem as enjoyable, but I can honestly say that come Monday morning I had no regrets. Also, the scale showed me a favorable number. It took two seasons for this habit to go away almost completely. Sometimes I still find myself craving an afternoon of mindless eating on game day, but I resist. It would not be worth the cost in calories or the disappointment in myself. It is paramount that in order to lose weight and keep it off, I had to make better choices, both short and long term. I also had to break the Sunday habit of saying, "I will begin a diet on Monday." I followed this habit for more years than I care to mention. Monday morning would arrive and nothing changed, resulting in a feeling of failure. No more.

The tools for success in changing my relationship with food:

- Developing a habit of not eating in social settings.

- Changing how I eat on game days or not eating at all.

- Keeping my favorite junk food out of the house—if you want it, you have to go get it.

- Get the people you live with on board with your new program.

- Recognize your food addictions and how they affect your weight and daily life.

- Look at this as changing your relationship with food. It is not a quick-fix diet.

- Take it one holiday at a time. You do not have to keep up unhealthy traditions. Start a new healthier tradition over time—slowly.

- Counting calories will keep you informed, aware and honest. It also creates a fantastic feeling of personal power.

- Read the labels of your favorite junk food and learn the hard truth about what you are putting into your body.

- Once you figure out your food addiction, slowly begin to eliminate it from your daily diet.

During my weight-loss journey, my eating habits slowly evolved from my old way of eating to a new, healthier lifestyle. As I weaned myself off of processed foods, I found myself craving healthier, simpler food. One of my favorite meals is a bowl of oatmeal with a banana and walnuts, along with some sort of protein like chicken or beef. If you asked me a year earlier would I enjoy this combination I would say, no way! I call it my one-ingredient lunch. Quaker oats, banana, walnuts, chicken, and beef all have one ingredient. There are no preservatives, chemicals or food coloring. It is also a very satisfying meal, and I usually have it for lunch. My energy level goes up rather than down following this meal.

Before I started eating Quaker oats, I was eating a packet of Trader Joe's Apple Cinnamon instant oatmeal. I liked it because it was portioned into a small envelope and it was 130 calories. One day I looked in the cabinet and there wasn't any instant oatmeal. There was a giant container of Quaker oats. I checked the ingredients and the calorie count and liked what I saw. I heated some up in the microwave. I was shocked at how bland it was compared to the instant oatmeal. I later looked at the ingredients in the instant oatmeal for the first time and saw that it was loaded with sugar and other additives. Before, I was just looking at the calorie count. Even though the Quaker oatmeal was bland, I continued to eat it and now I prefer it. I looked at this example of eating as an important lesson. I learned that I was open to evolving my eating habits over time and recognized that my tastes for certain foods and combinations changed to a more healthy and balanced way of eating. I was fueling my body with energy rather than filling my body with junk.

I still allow myself some sugary junk food twice a month, and I love it. My body does not. When I eat sugary, high fat or salty food, I immediately feel the difference in my energy level and disposition. It is the equivalent of a science experiment. Adding sugar and fat to my body changes the chemistry immediately. I pay the price in energy depletion and joint inflammation, resulting in sore knees, back and elbow joints. Eating sugar causes me to crash. It is almost not worth it. Someday, I hope to not even want these treat days. For now, I still enjoy these twice-monthly splurges even though the price is steep.

The cost may be high for my splurge days, but I consider them to be a key part of my success in keeping the weight off. If I can't have it, I want it. This is why quick-fix diets don't work.

Chapter Eight: *Sustainable Eating*

"Eat to live, don't live to eat."

–Benjamin Franklin

I have a confession to make: I never had a plan for what to eat except in the beginning, which was to cut out sugary junk food. Everything was based on this one decision for four months until I got the go-ahead from the doctor to get back to the gym, unrestricted. I didn't have a detailed plan or follow one of the popular diets. Those diets never worked for me. Why would I go that route again? During the three-month recovery I had plenty of time to think about the state of my life. I had a taste of not being able to walk, and I didn't like it. I also got to experience transporting my heavy body around on a walker, crutches and a cane. I really didn't like that either. I knew that opportunity was knocking, and that I really needed to open the door and make some very big changes in my life. What to do? What to do? I didn't do anything. I let things happen. First off, I knew it would take some time to lose all of the weight I had gained, so I decided to take the long view. I didn't put it on overnight and it sure wasn't coming off over-night either. I wanted this to be a lifestyle change. All of this would take time, and this was something new to me that I hadn't tried in the past. The idea of taking a year or longer to lose 80 pounds sounded right to me.

It also made sense. Another requirement that I had was that my diet had to be sustainable. What do I mean by that? I had to eat like I wasn't on a diet, with no feelings of deprivation or craving. The one non-negotiable rule was no sugary junk food. I just cannot eat this stuff on a regular basis. This may seem harsh to you, but I know me, and eating this food would lead me down the slippery path, and frankly, I like myself thin more than fat. Another Tony Robbins premise is that people will avoid pain more than they will seek out pleasure. I couldn't agree more. It may not be the same for you and that is okay.

Four months later I turned my attention to getting in shape with earnest and counting calories. I started to begin the process of elimination of foods I used to eat and began eating new foods that were satisfying and healthy. I did this very, very slowly. It took me three weeks to lose seven pounds. I had signed on to My Fitness Pal in November and that meant my first big challenge was the holidays. The beauty of it was now that I was counting calories: I was empowered with the knowledge of the calorie cost of a Thanksgiving and Christmas dinner. I still ate turkey, mashed potatoes, green beans and a dessert. I just didn't eat a lot. I knew that eating as much as I usually do during the holidays would set me back, and I had worked darn hard to lose those seven pounds. By the way, there were also two birthday celebrations in the month of December to contend with. This was my first and toughest challenge to date. I made it through the holidays with a three-pound weight loss. Once January 1, 2012 rolled around, I was on my way.

The following is a list of the foods that I eat regularly to this day.

- Stonyfield Low Fat Yogurt—I prefer this over Greek yogurt, and the extra 20 calories is worth the better taste value to me.

- Fruit, and that includes anything that is fresh and in season, such as apples, strawberries, raspberries, blueberries, pineapple, cantaloupe, pomegranates, plums, peaches, mangos and bananas.

- Almonds, walnuts.

- Lean protein—turkey, chicken, beef.

- Fresh homemade oatmeal bread.

- Wachusett potato chips, once or twice a week with a sandwich.

- Fresh vegetables—and that includes anything that is fresh and in season, such as English cucumbers, avocados, red and green peppers, all types of lettuces, onions, summer squash, zucchini and tomatoes.

- Fish—wild salmon, haddock, cod, halibut, swordfish—anything fresh and priced fairly.

- Peanut butter.

- Pasta—I limit my portion to one cup.

- Pizza, Janet's meatballs with tomato sauce.

- Beer, wine. I rarely drink hard liquor.

This is a sampling of what my daily diet consists of. I rarely drink any calories except when I have a glass of wine or beer. This is a huge calorie savings. When soft drinks first came out in the early part of the twentieth century, the normal size drink was six ounces. Today with everything super-sized, drinks range in size from 12 ounces to 64 ounces. That is a lot of useless, empty calories. I drink at least eight glasses of water per day, sometimes more. I do not drink diet soda. Diet soda is calorie free but not chemical free. Now that I pay close attention to what I am putting into my body, drinking something that has no nutritional value and is full of chemicals and additives is not an option.

It took almost a year to get to this point in what I eat. It may not look like much, but it is the norm for me now. I do go out to dinner every now and then, but because I changed my relationship with food, it doesn't come with the same anticipation as it used to. I choose restaurants known for the quality of their ingredients and creative menu. If you go to a restaurant and receive a heaping plate of food, and it is cheap, there is a reason for it—cheap inferior ingredients. It just isn't worth it to me anymore to eat junk.

Chapter Nine: *Feed Your Head*

"Many a small thing has been made large by the right kind of advertising."

–Mark Twain

We live in a society where a person's thinness and fitness determine an immediate judgment upon that individual. It isn't fair but it is true. The barometer for the reason for this unfairness begins and ends with our national obsession with being thin. This is ironic, because more than 45 percent of Americans are obese, yet we spend a lot of energy trying not to be.

Picture yourself wearing a hat with an antenna attached to it, sticking straight up into the sky. Every minute of every day you are receiving a broadcast of information in the form of advertisements and marketing, whether you are watching television, surfing the Internet, listening to the radio in your car or walking the aisles of the supermarket. No one has a chance of escaping this barrage unless you live on a deserted island out in the middle of the ocean without a wireless device. These are our times. The good news is that we can control our exposure to the marketing and advertisements by becoming more discerning about what we feed our head. What you feed your mind is just as important as what you physically put into your body. A steady diet of ad clicks, commercials and spam can be just as harmful as junk food eaten on a daily basis. It can undermine our efforts to not only lose weight but also anything we set out to accomplish. Hear me out.

When you log onto the Internet, the first page you see is your default browser, such as Safari, Internet Explorer, and Yahoo, to name a few. Unless you use a browser like Firefox, which has no ads or any distractions, you are exposed to a carefully laid out page that includes bits of news and hyperbole, along with advertisements and pop up banners sandwiched in between. With every page that you click to advertisers are looking for information about you and what your interests are. You may not pay attention to a lot of this consciously but it is subliminal and, whether you accept it or not, it is making its way into your subconscious. Information is what makes the Internet hum. The point I am trying to make is that we are human targets for marketers trying to get us to buy their products. This is nothing new. However, in the 21st century it has been turned into an art form online.

If you are going to establish a goal of losing weight, what you expose yourself to mentally is equally, if not more important, than what you actually eat. The mind is super powerful and can make or break your success in reaching your goal(s). That is why during my recovery period I had plenty of time to think and to come up with some very effective solutions for dealing with my lifelong struggle with food and losing weight. I avoided any and all media that highlighted food-related stories.

I created a very powerful tool that I used to help me reach my goal. When I first established a goal of losing 80 pounds, I decided to state to myself that I had already lost the weight. I would say, "I have lost 80 pounds and I weigh 110 pounds." This sends a message to your subconscious that you have created a new reality. Your subconscious then goes about making that new reality happen. If I said, "I will lose 80 pounds," it sends the message that the goal *will always be in the future and will never happen*. Once I made this statement, I reinforced it with a strong belief in myself that it **would** happen.

How do you get yourself into a state of believing? I repeated the statement "I have lost 80 pounds and I weigh 110 pounds," over and over. I found a photo of myself when I had weighed 110 pounds and propped it up against my computer where I would see it constantly. Every time I sat at my computer I saw that photo; it reminded me that I weighed 110 pounds. The combination of a clearly stated goal said in the present tense, reinforced with a photo, works like magic. This is a perfect example of feeding your head in a positive way.

I took this concept one step further by recording positive clear statements in my own voice. I used a small digital recorder and then downloaded the audio file onto the iPod in my iPhone. Before I went to sleep at night I would listen to these statements on a loop until I dropped off into a deep sleep. Everything was stated as if it already happened. This is a very effective and powerful way of getting yourself into a state of believing for achieving any goal. Here are samples of what I was telling myself.

- I have lost 80 pounds and I weigh 110 pounds.

- I am super fit.

- I am successful, positive, loving and kind.

- I eat like a normal person.

- I am getting stronger every day.

A super fit mind goes hand in hand with a super fit body; you can't have one without the other. What you feed your head matters.

Chapter Ten:
What You Look Like Matters

"I think perfect objectivity is an unrealistic goal;
fairness, however, is not."

–Michael Pollan

In a perfect world everyone would accept one another for who they are and what they look like. Unfortunately, this isn't always the case. I am going to go out on a limb and state that overweight people are treated differently, sometimes unfairly and sometimes by other overweight people. Most of the time you do not know you are being judged. Privately, we are all insecure, especially about how we look and how much extra weight we are carrying around. I have friends who are super skinny and deathly afraid of gaining weight. These same friends look down their noses at those folks who are overweight. Even if a person is thin or of average weight they still share the same feelings of shame and self-loathing as those who are overweight. Do you get my drift?

According to a study done by George Washington University in 2010, "An overweight individual will make up to 15% less than their equally educated and experienced colleague. The overweight individual will pay an additional $2,646.00 per year in direct costs if male and $4,879.00 if female. They will take more time off from work than their normal-weight colleague; they are less likely to be hired and more quickly to be let go."

Wow! Being overweight is not only unhealthy, but it also costs you money! If your employer is constantly looking at the bottom line, which is what businesses do, they do not want to hire you if you are overweight, believing, correctly, that it will cost them more money. When promotions or opportunities for advancement come up, the odds are that it will go to your thin colleague who has the same resume and experience. This doesn't seem fair, but as your mother told you early on, life isn't always fair. The truth hurts, but knowledge is power. Knowing that these biases exist could serve as a great motivator for beginning the quest to lose weight. If saving money is the deal breaker for making big changes in your life, then so be it. Whatever it takes to get you up off the couch and away from the refrigerator—great! This is good news because all of this is avoidable.

I cannot tell you how many times people have complimented me on losing the pounds. Total strangers have come up to me on the street and told me how proud they are of me because I had lost weight. Nobody came up to me when I was *morbidly obese* and complimented me about my weight. Now that I weigh 110 pounds I am treated much differently—all of it in a good way. It is because I am thin, happier and give off a good vibe. I feel like I hit the lottery. I can buy clothes that are in single-digit sizes instead of one-size fits all. My health has improved. I am no longer at risk for all sorts of chronic illnesses. Losing the weight has given me a fighting chance at optimum health. My metabolism has increased. There is no downside to losing weight.

I gained weight slowly over 12 years. If you eat just 20 extra calories a day you will gain an additional 21 pounds over a ten-year period. No wonder I gained eighty pounds. I had a lot of fun along the way but I paid a high cost. Which is why I will never go back to where I was before. I love being thin more than I want to eat a diet of unhealthy and fattening foods. I want to maintain my weight and enjoy the multitude of benefits that come with it rather than pick up my old eating habits. It is work, though. Maintaining my weight requires constant vigilance. I continue to log what I eat into My Fitness Pal every day. I always stay within my calorie allotment. I had a base of 1330 calories while I was losing weight. My maintenance number is 1590 calories per day. This is only an increase of 260 calories. I get on the scale at least once a week. I work out hard six to seven days per week. I use the extra calories that I burn during my workout, adding them on to my 1590-calorie allotment. I use a heart rate monitor to measure my calories for workouts other than my Arc Trainer sessions. What I am getting at here is that once I reached my goal, life did not change. I eat the same foods, and depending on how hungry I am, I may eat more of them. My sugar addiction still follows me around wherever I go. I allow myself two treat days per month. Notice, I didn't say cheat days. This is dangerous territory because my brain wants another sugar fix the next day. It is almost not worth it. I do not drink alcohol a lot because it leads to bad choices. Drinking erases all reason and logic, and you end up at some late night burger joint that also serves giant desserts. I do not overindulge when I enjoy a drink or two. I stay away from white wine and hard liquor, especially vodka. I usually stick to a glass of red wine or beer.

Initially, my catalyst for losing weight was because of the repercussions that evolved from breaking my leg. My life literally came to a screeching halt. Not being able to walk, work or drive really made an impression on me. The total recovery period ended up taking more than eight months. My ankle works well, but for every step I take I can feel the presence of those eleven pins and two plates that hold my right ankle together. I feel fortunate to live in the 21st century where medicine and technology meet at the crossroads for healing not just a broken leg, but also an endless array of illnesses and injuries. I am not going to minimize my injury, but I am also aware that what happened to me wasn't life threatening. I did not have a near-death experience where I saw the light and came back appreciating that what really matters is living a great and loving life. I already live a great and loving life. I did open the door when opportunity came knocking. I made choices that would help me reach all of my goals. I believe that once you reach a goal you need to have a few more ready to go. Goals are dreams that come true. When I started my weight-loss journey, trying to lose weight seemed like the impossible dream. It was like trying to get back to the island and forgetting how to swim.

We live in a time when we do not have to hunt or forage for our food to survive. All we have to do is walk through the doors of the local supermarket where there is an endless array of foods. According to Wikipedia, the definition of food is, "any substance consumed to provide nutritional support for the body."

A lot of crunchy snacks do not fall into the food category. Reading and understanding the list of ingredients on the back of a bag of your favorite salty snack requires a degree in food science. Years ago, I was visiting my brother in Florida. He was a chef and taught a class at a local community college on how to make Danish and other assorted desserts. I went along with him on one of his class nights. I was training for the Big Sur Marathon at the time and was abstaining from desserts. On the drive over we were talking about frosting (natch) and how it was made. The ingredients are lard and sugar! I love supermarket cakes with lots of frosting, especially the corners with roses and extra piping. When he told me the truth about frosting, it was a huge letdown. I never thought about what went into the making of frosting. And that's the problem; I never took the time to think about it. I did not want to know how junk food is made. If people really thought about what those crunchy snacks are made of, they would think twice before opening the bag. Ignorance is bliss until we add on a few pounds and feel awful both physically and mentally later on.

When entering a supermarket, you should prepare for sensory overload, especially if you are hungry. It is a marketing and advertising war zone. You have no chance if you allow yourself to be seduced by the sights, sounds, flashy displays, colorful packaging and smells from the bakery—that is usually located near the front entrance. The food industry spends millions on marketing and advertising, all aimed at getting us to buy their products. The negotiations between vendors and stores for prime product placement on shelves would have made Tony Soprano envious. In other words, you are a target the moment you enter the building. I am not criticizing the free enterprise system, but if you want to change your relationship with food in order to lose weight, you must develop a keen awareness of your marketing and advertising vulnerabilities. Pretty much everything that is unprocessed and healthy is available on the outside aisles, such as fresh produce and dairy and protein sources like meat, fish and poultry. Start moving to the center and you come face first with the snack and cookie aisles, along with every other processed food product available. Always eat before you shop to eliminate unwanted temptation. It is a good idea to go in with a game plan to go along with your shopping list.

There is a term called "clean eating" that is popular today. According to fitness guru, Tony Horton of P90X fame, it means eating foods that have no preservatives, additives or chemicals in the ingredient list. If there is a mysterious ingredient you can't pronounce or if it evokes an image of guys in white lab coats, you probably shouldn't be eating it. He also talks about the 90-10 rule: The idea that you should stick to eating clean foods 90% of the time instead of 100%. This rule is important because we all need to include some treat days and meals in our diets to allow us to reward ourselves and to keep us on track.

Eating clean should be slowly integrated into your diet over time. When I started my journey, I eliminated sugary junk food and anything with corn syrup added to it. Other than this first step everything else was literally on the table. My plan was to do this gradually and through a process of elimination. I could never go from the way I was eating to a diet that was so radically different. This would have automatically set me up for failure—again.

Chapter Eleven:
The Gift That Keeps On Giving

"Miracles come in moments.
Be ready and willing."
—Wayne Dyer

Breaking my leg in the summer of 2011 has truly been the gift that keeps on giving. I believe the operative word is "BREAKING." I wanted to make big changes in my life a year before my accident, but my work as a freelance photojournalist got in the way. Even though I loved my job, I was ready for a change. Then the universe stepped in and made some decisions for me. I believe when you ask for change the universe presents opportunities and choices in subtle, unexpected ways. I got distracted when this happened to me, and I ignored the opportunities and experiences instead of seeing them for what they were. I wanted change, but I kept taking assignments for the money instead of answering my calling. Fast-forward to July 2, 2011, and the universe decided for me. If I wasn't going to take the necessary steps to make the changes I wanted and asked for then I would get literal and figurative help. So what if I broke my leg in three places? I wanted to make three major changes and the price was breaking three bones in my right leg. It has been worth every moment and more.

The three changes I asked for were to lose all of the weight I had gained over a 12-year period, write a book and develop a public speaking career. Today, I can say, mission accomplished. It took me almost two years to reach these goals but I did. I am living proof that anybody can make a change(s) in their life at any time or any age if they believe they can and focus like a laser beam on what they want to achieve. As the great motivational speaker, Napoleon Hill famously stated, "What the mind of a man can conceive and believe, it can achieve." How true! The only limitations we have are those that we put in front of ourselves.

Not too long ago I was walking out of my local library and across the parking lot to my car when I heard someone calling out to me, trying to get my attention. It was a woman who I have seen over the years at various events and places but we never really had a real conversation or exchanged first names. Her name is Clair, I have come to find out. Clair got my attention and asked if I went through a year of transformation. Clair also works at the gym where I had my previous membership. The last time she saw me I had spent three months weaning myself off of my crutches and cane. Also, I was 60 pounds heavier. We chatted awhile and I filled her in on how I went about my transformation, and then I thanked her for noticing. Clair exclaimed enthusiastically, "How could I not?" I got into my car feeling proud, peaceful and happy with my accomplishment.

The next day while walking my dog along my street, a neighbor who I see all of the time but with whom I had never had any communication, was barreling down the street on his Harley Davidson motorcycle. He yelled out to me, "Looking good!" I yelled back, "Thanks!" These are the little miracles that come from making a profound change in your life. You don't think people are paying attention, but they are. I learned that of the three goals I set out for myself, the one I always get asked about is, "How did you lose the weight?" I believe a majority of the population is challenged with being overweight and everyone desperately wants to be thin and healthy. I am no different. That day I picked up my medical records and read that I was listed as being *morbidly obese* got my attention. I felt shame and hopelessness. However, it still took me six months and a broken leg to do something about it. As I lost weight over the year, I passed from being *morbidly obese*, to obese, to overweight, and finally, to normal weight. Each passage was a milestone, taking me one step closer to my current reality.

Even now I can't believe I had weighed 190 pounds. Setting the table for success required many tools, including getting clear on my goals and establishing a simple plan with three components to assist me in reaching my goal. I believe that taking the long view and deciding to change my relationship with food was a critical first step in losing 80 pounds. Counting calories and using My Fitness Pal was hugely important to my success and continues to be to this day. Counting calories is 80% part and parcel to losing and maintaining weight. The exercise workouts are the other 20% and are important, but for different reasons. A person who goes to the gym and works out on the Elliptical machine for thirty minutes might burn three hundred calories. Following the workout they stop at the local coffee shop and buy a "healthy" blueberry muffin that has 600 calories and a large coffee with cream and sugar (100 calories). The total calorie intake is 700 calories and that is just breakfast. There is a 400-calorie differential that eventually catches up to us over time with a weight gain. Change out the muffin for a half a cup of low fat yogurt and a half cup of fresh blueberries and you are right around 100 calories. That is a huge difference! Now there is a 200-calorie credit in your daily energy bank, and the day is still young. The muffin sounds more appealing until you remember how hard you worked out on the Elliptical machine. Therein lies the rub. It is all about choices. You can go to the gym every day and workout, but if you don't put the fork down and think about what you are feeding your body, successful weight loss will elude you. Working out for an hour a day is great, but the real challenge is the food choices you make during the remaining 23 hours that will make or break weight loss success.

Junk food is created to make you addicted and to make you want to crave the sugary or salty snacks to keep you reaching for more. There is no redeeming nutritional value in junk food, including soda. I found that as time passed and I slowly eliminated certain foods from my daily diet the desire quieted down. Being able to say no to bad food in the moment and make better choices is available to us all. Is it a sacrifice? Sometimes. The times when I am tempted I hang in there and wait, and boy, I am always glad I did. Coincidently, drinking alcohol makes me make bad food choices. Why wouldn't it? You are literally not in your right mind. I still have a glass of wine or an occasional beer, knowing the risk. I eat potato chips with a sandwich. Also, I eat pizza once a week. The difference is that I always stay within my daily calorie allotment. I log into My Fitness Pal every day and record every single thing I eat. It keeps me honest and on track and it is easy. What I am trying to say is that maintaining my weight will always be a challenge to me, and I accept this fact. I enjoy life and never feel like I am on a diet. If I did think I was on a diet it would never have worked. I tell myself every day that I eat like a normal person, and I do.

During the summer of 2011, while I was using a walker and crutches as my main source of transportation, I had many experiences that would add up to what I will call my Ebenezer Scrooge moments. Ebenezer Scrooge was the main character in, *A Christmas Carol*, by Charles Dickens.[1] While dreaming one night he had three visitors—the past, the present and the future. Each visitor took him on a tour of his life from each vantage point. I am not saying I had the exact same experience, but I do feel that while recovering from my accident, I had plenty of time to think about my past, present and future.

I knew that by being *morbidly obese* I was really unhappy and uncomfortable in so many ways. I had no agility and was often out of breath if I exerted myself in any way. Running down the sidelines of a football field carrying 20 pounds of camera gear was tough going. I had the photojournalist mentality—get the shot, no matter what. I would put myself in situations that I would pay for later. I climbed scaffolding, crawled onto rooftops, drove through Nor'easter's looking for accidents and downed trees, and got hit by hockey pucks—you name it; I would get the shot and do it without fear. One of the editors often referred to me as the intrepid photographer—fearless. When I would arrive home from a day of assignments I would be sore and tired but happy with my photos. My chiropractor would say to me, "Oh, your poor neck!" because I carried my Nikon D3 with a large zoom lens attached to it around my neck. I never thought of my physical limitations when going for the shot. As I said earlier, my uniform for six years was my synthetic work-out pants—one size fits all—and a large T-shirt. Up until this point I hadn't found a good reason to change my life until I broke my leg and life came to a screeching halt.

During the summer months after my injury we went out a few times to restaurants, stores and other places and quickly learned what life is like as a handicapped person. My physical therapist, Susan, suggested that swimming would accelerate the healing process. I had to buy a bathing suit, which in itself was a humiliating experience. I arrived at a local sporting goods store prepared to shop for a bathing suit and found the front electric doors not operating. According to the sales clerk they were turned off to save money. The clerk had to hold the door open for me so I could hobble in. Because it was October in New England, bathing suits were on display at the furthest corner of the large box store. I persevered and after the horror of trying a bathing suit on in the dressing room I made the purchase. I made a mental note and added another link to the growing list of reasons to lose weight. When I saw my reflection in the dressing room mirror I asked myself again, "How did this happen?" Dressing room mirrors are unforgiving.

My first trip to the pool was arduous. I had to get into the building on my crutches, make my way to the locker room, change into my suit, shower and then make my way to the far end of the pool where the ramp was so that I could grab onto the railing and gradually make my way down the ramp and into the pool. Every step took three times the effort it would if I could walk on two legs.

My past was being grotesquely overweight, my present was filled with opportunity and choices, and my future would be the results from those choices. I could remain the same—playing Russian roulette with my health and staying in a dead-end career—or I could take the path that would lead me to a healthier life and a promising career as an author and professional speaker. I chose the latter.

I had my Ebenezer moments through my daily experiences. I knew at age 55 that I was tempting fate—and not the kind I wanted. I wanted to lose the weight for reasons of vanity, but I was also acutely aware that I was at an age where health issues could threaten, not only the quality of my life, but also my life itself. I now had a reason to believe. I got very clear on what I wanted to do and this decision alone put me on the path to reaching my goal of losing 80 pounds, writing this book and becoming a super successful public speaker.

I had lots of aches and pains that I chalked up to carrying my camera gear. In 2009, I had arthroscopic surgery on my left knee. My knees always hurt. I couldn't stand for long periods of time because my back would hurt. I thought, well, that is what it is like when you hit middle age. Yes and no. Because I was carrying so much weight, not eating right and not doing any kind of workout program, everything was going to hell in a handbasket. My body was breaking down because I wasn't taking care of it. We take better care of our cars and homes than we do ourselves. Everyone and everything else comes first. Guess what? If we do not take care of ourselves first we will be in no position to care for others, especially those we love.

Now let's talk about the good news. The human body is incredibly resilient and forgiving! Given the right food and exercise you can turn that car wreck into a Ferrari, even at this stage of the game. I am living proof! Presently, I am in better shape than I was as a marathon runner. I ran a lot! However, I did not do any strength or conditioning exercise. I had very little upper-body strength. Today, I have overall total body strength. I can do pushups, lift weights, and I have a strong core! I am literally a new person!

In little more than one year I managed, through a lot of hard work and discipline, to transform my body to one that is high energy, slim and healthy. Life became exponentially easier and more satisfying. The message here is that although we are on the other side of 50 that doesn't mean we have to be soft with no muscle tone and low energy. Perhaps it is characteristic of the baby boomer generation that we want to hold onto youthful, healthy bodies. I say, so what, to that! I am a boomer and I want to be able to move with ease and purpose over the next few decades. I want to give myself the best possible advantage to be as fit and healthy as possible. And while I am at it, I want to look good and feel vibrant and alive.

People say they don't have time to exercise. Really? I found this quote by Edward Stanley, Earl of Derby in 1873:

"Those who think they have not time for bodily exercise will sooner or later have to find time for illness."

Edward Stanley was a forward thinker in his day. This quote caught my eye because a lot of people use the excuse that they do not have time for exercise. I am not casting aspersions here because I am guilty of the same behavior. Remember, before I broke my leg I had a gym membership that I used for a month and then quit because I didn't like it or didn't have the time. Not only did I quit going to the gym, I also didn't do much else besides the exercise I got from working and the occasional walk. This was the behavior of a former marathon runner? Unfortunately, that is what my lifestyle morphed into over a 12-year period.

Lately, I find my conversations with some people include talking about aches and pains, doctor's visits and the aging process. How depressing is this? Are you one of those people who spend a lot of time in doctor's offices? You may not want to be there but you make the time. If we do not take care of our body's health issues, spending precious time in hospital waiting rooms will become reality.

Once women turn 50 their metabolism slows down due to the natural aging process. According to the University of California, Los Angeles, Student Nutrition Awareness Campaign (SNAC), "As you lose muscle mass, gain fat mass and experience hormonal changes, your resting metabolic rate, which accounts for 65% of your daily calorie burn, will decrease. By age 50 your metabolism will be 10-20% lower than in your 20s and 30s."[2] The good news is that by putting yourself through a strenuous workout that includes not only cardio but also free weights, you can raise your metabolism by building new muscle tissue and promote new cell growth. This is imperative as we get older.

My workout time each day is non-negotiable. I always work out in the morning; otherwise, life gets in the way, creating a thousand excuses not to exercise. It is as important to me as taking a shower and brushing my teeth, which I would never skip. I feel I owe it to myself to put my body through the paces because the advantages outweigh the disadvantages. If I can possibly avoid spending time in doctor's offices and hospitals, I will do whatever it takes. That means making it to my workout appointment each and every day. I consider my workouts to be a part of my job. My brother, Joey, once said to me. "An hour or more working out each day is a small investment of time." He was right!

We only have so much time here and I want to make the most of each and every day. By taking care of my body—my Ferrari—it will take care of me.

Chapter Twelve: *The Personal Toolbox*

"We become what we behold. We shape our own tools, and thereafter our tools shape us."

– Marshall McLuhan

O nce I got myself to the starting line of this journey I knew that I would be using a variety of tools to help me along the way. I refer to this as my personal toolbox. Some of the tools were intangible, such as decisiveness, perseverance, discipline and maintaining a positive mental attitude. These tools come from within. Then there are the tangible tools that are actually something you can hold in your hand. I will highlight some of the tools here and demonstrate how effective they were in assisting me in reaching the goals I set for myself.

Photographs

I am deeply moved by photographs. I understand the power behind a meaningful photo. Visualization is a powerful intangible tool and when there is a photo to back up the visualization process, massive change is not only possible but also inevitable.

A few weeks after I returned to the gym, I dug deep into my archives for a photo of myself that I liked before I gained all the weight. There were not many to choose from. I never wanted my photo to be taken, especially from the neck down. I found one of me taken in 1994, rowing a boat on a lake in New Hampshire. I was thin and in shape, having run the Boston Marathon the previous April. I took this photo and propped it up against my iMac alongside the X-ray of my ankle with all 11 pins and two plates showing. By doing this I was reinforcing my goal of weighing 110 pounds as if it had already happened. Every time I sat down at my computer I looked at the picture.

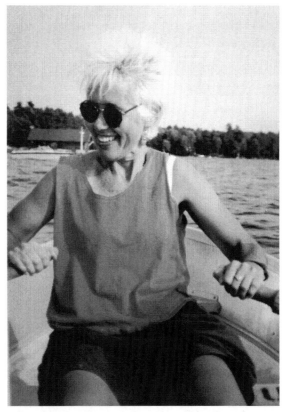

Me, before the weight gain. This photo was an inspiration to reach my weight loss goal.

I used the rowing photo as a present-tense photo. I would say to myself, "I weigh 110 pounds or less," even though I was quite a ways from this number. I said this to myself as if it was already true. I got myself into a state of believing and then let it go. I am always at my computer and the photo served me well. Most times I didn't consciously think about the photo, even though I looked at it on average of 40 to 50 times a day. It became a subliminal message over time. It was my own personal advertising and marketing campaign. The image kept flashing across my brain, paving the way to my new reality.

The photo of my leg X-ray served as a reminder of how far I had come since the accident and how fortunate I was to be able to walk again. The X-ray photo, in my opinion, was the most compelling photo of 2011. When I show it to people they either cringe or appreciate the medical wizardry that went into making my right leg and foot work almost seamlessly together again. I believe the constant presence of this photo assisted in the healing process on a deeply subconscious level.

Using photos as a tool to achieve a goal, especially a weight-loss goal, can be one of the most tangible tools in your toolbox. It was in mine.

HRM
(Heart Rate Monitor)

Based on my strong belief that counting calories is the most effective way to lose the pounds, using a heart rate monitor is an especially powerful tool to have in the toolbox. Using a heart rate monitor tells you many things, but most importantly, it counted my exercise calories. I used a heart rate monitor when I began my first round of the boot camp program P90X. It wasn't necessary to use an HRM at the gym because the read-out on the Arc Trainer kept me informed of how many calories I burned during a session. I always burned way more calories on the Arc Trainer than I did during my P90X workouts. This is why I continued to use the Arc Trainer even though I added P90X to my daily workouts in early April. I needed to know how many calories I was burning so that I could add them to my numbers in My Fitness Pal. If I burned 500 calories on the Arc Trainer and another 300 doing one of the P90X DVDs, that adds up to 800 calories that I added onto my daily allotted 1330 calories. This is a significant number because now I am up to 2130 calories so far for the day. I rarely would eat these calories back, so it actually accelerated my weight loss.

I use a Polar HRM, but there are many heart rate monitors to choose from. If I had a suggestion for the companies who make heart rate monitors it would be to offer different sizes for the chest strap. By the time I reached my goal I had stapled and duct-taped my chest strap so it would stay on properly. It wasn't a bad problem to have because it was another way of measuring my progress. It would be more convenient and comfortable to have a different size with an adjustable chest strap.

I use my HRM when I go on vacation. This might seem a bit obsessive to some people but not me. We all know that when we go on vacation or a long weekend away all hell breaks loose in the eating department. We feel like we have a green light to eat anything and everything we want because we are living outside our daily routine. This can be costly—like a five-pound weight gain costly. I would rather know how many calories I burned and have a reference point to work with than throw the baby out with the bath water and not care. You can indulge but within reason. Let's face it; I worked too hard to get rid of the weight only to gain some back because I was on vacation. This is a lifestyle change and that includes when on vacation or special occasions such as birthdays and holidays.

I spent a few days in Maine last summer and wore my HRM constantly. I went on a hike and burned 800-plus calories. I kept on the move and earned some extra calories so I could indulge a bit at dinner. This is just self-discipline through management of calories whenever and wherever you find yourself. I never regret staying within my daily calorie allotment. Actually, I feel empowered and quite happy with myself. I always remind myself that this is a lifestyle change and a major shift in my relationship with food.

My heart rate monitor was money well spent. I encourage anyone traveling the weight loss journey to purchase one. My HRM is tired looking these days, but it still keeps chugging along, counting my calories. One footnote to counting calories, as you lose weight your body burns calories more efficiently. A workout I did with an extra 40 or 50 pounds burned more calories than I do today at my current weight of 110 pounds. It is a happy adjustment.

Free Weights

I started using free weights during the time I began P90X. Today I use them almost exclusively for my strength training. Pushing and pulling weight is an old-fashioned and effective way to develop muscle tissue. When I started out, I used three-pound weights and over time increased the weight as I became stronger and fit. The feeling of strength, particularly in your shoulders and arms, is particularly gratifying.

As we grow older, developing new muscle tissue is critical to a healthy aging process. Once we hit 50 and over our metabolisms slow down and we become less active. This is a deadly combination. To combat the effects of aging, even healthy aging, it is imperative to develop strength and move more. Otherwise, our bodies turn to mush. Men and women entering their fifties and beyond tend to have bodies that are not toned or muscular. It is like we give up on believing that you can have a hard, muscular fit body well into old age. Remember the fitness guru, Jack Lalanne? This guy was so far ahead of his time. He began eating healthy and lifting weights back in the 1930s. They say he was working out right up until the day before he died at the age of 95 years old. Using free weights or weight machines is part of the answer to healthy aging.

I use the free weights at my local gym because I have outgrown the weights that I have at home. I have gone from using three-pound weights up to 15, 20 and 25-pound weights for certain exercises. I use barbells for squats, toe raises, overhead presses and bench presses. My transition from having very little muscle strength didn't happen overnight. It has taken me more than a year of consistently using free weights, barbells and cardio exercise to achieve the level of fitness that I now enjoy. Muscle tissue growth happens slowly over time, much to the frustration of skinny teenage boys. The only ones developing big muscles over a short period of time are taking supplements that are detrimental to their health.

My daily workouts now are different from a year ago. I go to the gym and use the Arc Trainer for 50-60 minutes and average a calorie burn of somewhere between 600-800 calories. I follow this up with 20-30 minutes of free weight training, depending on which group of muscles I am working that day. When I get home I make sure to do 30-40 pushups. Even I am impressed that I can do that many pushups.

Lifting, pushing and pulling weights, as Dr. Jonathan Sullivan states, "Is good medicine." I really push myself hard and lift enough weight that pushes me beyond my current level of fitness. It is the only way to become stronger. Strength training with free weights and barbells is hard work that pays infinite dividends.

The Arc Trainer

The cardio part of my workout is done on the Arc Trainer. The Arc trainer is a machine made by Cybex. I use the Arc trainer at my gym five or six days a week, depending on my energy level. I discovered this machine while perusing the success stories category in the community section of My Fitness Pal. A woman was telling her story about how she successfully reached her weight-loss goal. She mentioned the Arc Trainer, and how many calories she was able to burn during her workout—700! I knew right then and there that I had to start using the Arc trainer. This machine is similar to an elliptical machine but is a better calorie burner. According to the Cybex website, using the Arc trainer burns 16% more calories than the elliptical. This is because it works the large muscles of both the hips and the knees. I was sold. Because I can no longer run marathons or run very far, very often, my time on the Arc trainer has replaced running for me. It is low impact and loosens my ankle up every day. It also adds up to a 700 plus additional calorie burn each day. As you probably have surmised, when I go to the gym, I am all business. Sometimes I see people arrive at the gym with a large coffee and a newspaper. I guess it is better than doing nothing, but I like to get the most bang for my buck while working out.

When I first started using the Arc trainer, I could go only fifteen minutes at level ten, which was challenging but doable. Overtime, I have worked my way up to level 32 for 50-60 minutes, depending on the day. My blood pressure and resting heartbeat numbers are excellent, and I attribute this to my time on the Arc trainer and, of course, being 80 pounds lighter.

The Arc trainer isn't for everyone but it has and continues to serve me well. There are those who want to de-emphasize calorie burning, especially spending time on the "road to nowhere," but it is a matter of preference and works for me.

P90X

In 2010, I bought the boot camp program P90X on EBay. I was impressed with the infomercial featuring Tony Horton, the face of P90X, and what he had to say. There were a lot of testimonials that were convincing as well. When I received the box in the mail, I quickly realized that this program was too much for me to handle. I didn't even open the box. I put it away until April 2012, when I weighed 148 pounds and had been working out for five full months and felt like I could handle the program. I decided to commit to the first round of the program no matter what. My copy of the program, which I purchased on EBay, didn't include the nutrition guide or the book on how to use the program. No wonder it was so cheap. There are 12 DVDs in the box, each one devoted to a different set of muscles and other workouts. One day you might be working on your chest and back, and the next day doing an hour of plyometrics or jump training. Because I didn't have the books I just did each DVD one after another. This turned out to be dumb luck because doing it this way eased me into the program. I was only a little more than half way to my weight-loss goal and I was wary about how far I could push my now-healed ankle.

The first 90-day round went like that and when I began round two, I smartened up. Some friends that I knew who were also doing the program lent me their books, and I began to follow the program the correct way. They said that I would see results right away and they were right. All in all, I did four rounds of P90X over the year. There is nothing negative about this program. If you do the work consistently the results are fantastic. If you cannot do what Tony and his crew are doing in the video, you modify the exercise until you can. I started out doing all of the pushups on my knees (girl pushups). The program has you doing a multitude of pushups of every variety. The only pushups I could never do off my knees were the one hand behind my back and the clappers. I can live with this. Today, I can do 40-50 pushups. It is hard but the feeling afterward is magical.

These days I have streamlined my workouts from two hours per day to 70-90 minutes per day at the gym. This may sound like a large commitment, but it is time well spent and well worth it.

Scales

There are two types of scales that I use, one for weighing food portions and one for weighing myself. I continue to weigh most everything I eat. Doing this keeps me informed about the amount of calories I am eating in relation to the number of calories I am burning. Knowledge is power! Increasing your calories consistently over your daily allotment, even by 10 or 20 calories over a period of years, results in a steady and quiet weight gain. One day you wake up, and surprise, you have 20 extra pounds to deal with. I know, because this is how I found myself in the predicament of being 80 pounds overweight. The difference was that I was eating a heck of a lot more than 10 or 20 extra calories per day. Long-term weight gain sneaks up on you, and one day you look in the mirror and find yourself to be *morbidly obese* like I was. The good news is that this theory works conversely. If you eliminate 10-20 calories each day over a long period you will lose weight without even trying. Today, the food scale is and always will be an important tool in my personal toolbox.

The other scale is the one I avoided for a decade. I never wanted to know how much I weighed because I knew that I was heading into dangerous waters, and in my case it was the river of denial. I remember going to the doctor for my annual physical in January 2011, getting on the scale and telling the nurse—as I looked away—not to tell me the number. I learned a year and a half later that I weighed 190 pounds. The following year, I was in for another physical and I told the nurse I had lost 42 pounds and she said, "No, you have lost 50 pounds." I was stunned. Now I weigh myself a minimum of once a week, sometimes twice. Again, knowledge is power! My weight fluctuates from week to week. Some days I weigh 108 and other days I weigh 110 pounds. I try to never go above 110 pounds. This is the line in the sand for me.

I do not fear the scale anymore. I use it for what it is, a tool to measure how much I weigh. It gives a number to work with and helps keep me honest with myself.

Recording Device

I am a believer in the power of positive affirmations. I am not talking about taping little yellow post-it notes to my bathroom mirror. That works for some people, but I like to take it a step further. During my weight loss journey, I recorded, in my own voice, a series of affirmations or statements regarding my goals. I always state my affirmations in the present tense. I used a little digital recorder and then downloaded the audio files into iTunes and then onto my iPhone. I am sure there are apps that you can download directly into your Smartphone, but this is the method I used. Before I went to sleep at night I would put my headphones on and lull myself to sleep hearing my voice repeat positive affirmations over and over again. I guess you could say I bored myself to sleep—in a good way. Here is a sampling of some of the affirmations that I used.

-I weigh 110 pounds.

-I eat like a normal person.

-I am strong and fit.

-I wear awesome-fitting jeans.

-The pounds continue to melt away each and every day.

-I am healthy.

I listened to myself making these statements on a continuous loop each night for months. The messages seeped into my subconscious mind, and over time, became real to me. I believe in this method 100 percent. Being aware of the power of your subconscious, both in a positive and negative way, is important. The power of suggestion works for and against you when on the quest for reaching any and all goals. Obviously, you want to take the positive route, while being mindful of any negative energy around you.

These are the tangible tools that I use in my personal toolbox. They have served me well. Perhaps they might help you on your quest for losing weight or any type of Self-improvement goal.

Chapter Thirteen: *Time Well Spent*

**"They always say time changes things, but you
actually have to change them yourself."**

–Andy Warhol

On October 15, 2012, I reached my original goal weight of 115 pounds. The day after, the sun rose in the east and nothing changed for me. I ate the same foods, worked out the same way and logged into My Fitness Pal. A few weeks went by and I continued to lose weight. Toward the end of November I had lost eight more pounds. That is pretty thin, even for a shorty like me. According to the Center for Disease Control Body Mass Index,[1] I was well within normal range for a person of my height and weight. When I started out on this journey I was *morbidly obese* and weighed in at a whopping 190 pounds. I lost a total of 83 pounds in a little over a year. That is the weight of your average sixth grader. My dog, Bandit, weighs 86 pounds. I lost the weight of a whole person or a large dog.

The fact that life did not change on October 16th, 2012, is exactly the way I wanted it to be. This is a lifestyle change, not a quick fix or a temporary way of living and eating. Eating right and working out hard are a way of life for me now. I never, ever, want to be overweight again. The initial motivation for losing weight began when I broke my leg and realized how hard it was to get around on crutches or using a walker carrying 80 extra pounds. However, over time it evolved into a much larger issue for me. I realized at age 55 that I was now on the other side of middle age and things were not looking very promising. I was on the cusp of developing a chronic illness or worse if I did not choose to take a different path. Once I stated my goals I got to work. Getting to where I am now required patience, perseverance, focus and self-discipline, all useful tools that can be used for any kind of goal attainment. I learned that change, real lasting change, takes time and effort. I realized that the days of overeating and not getting enough exercise was over if I wanted to maintain this fantastic fitness level.

My new goal is to keep myself at my optimum weight, work out hard and position myself for a long and healthy aging process. I want to stay healthy for as long as I can, so that when my health declines, it will hopefully happen when I am very old. I am not naive in thinking that I won't get sick or meet an untimely end before becoming elderly, but at least I can do everything in my power to set myself up for success and a high quality of life for as long as possible.

As a baby boomer, I am acutely aware that the next 20 years are going to bring massive changes to our healthcare system. Without getting into details about the Affordable Care Act, it is safe to say that health care as we know it will be very different.

Medicare, believe it or not, is a very streamlined operation. Program managers assign a certain amount of money per procedure and rarely if ever deviate from this policy. Already doctors are turning away Medicare patients because the money is to be made elsewhere. This is the new reality. The great news is that taking responsibility for your lifestyle and getting as healthy as possible will lessen the effect of the health-care industry on your life. The high costs of the baby boomer generation entering retirement age will come to pass over the next 20 years, if not sooner.

Why am I even writing about this? If you are over 50 and overweight, this information directly affects you. A friend of mine asked me, "What is the value that readers will take away from reading your book?" The obvious one is that my story of losing close to 50 percent of my body weight and becoming super fit in the process might inspire folks to think about improving their health. Stories are important to me. Nobody wants to be told what to do or be lectured. There are no charts, graphs or a bunch of statistics in this book to make your eyes glaze over. That kind of information is all over the Internet, in books and periodicals. This is real life. I am an expert on me changing my life. I am not exceptional or athletically gifted. I am like you. If you can take one or two things from this book and it helps you to change your life, then writing this book is a huge success.

Stories are more interesting than someone telling you to follow a plan starting with A and getting to Z. I make suggestions, but in reality how and why you change your life is up to you. It is personal, customized and unique.

The value is showing you by example that making positive changes in your life, whether it be losing weight, quitting smoking or beginning a workout program, is not only worth the effort but also could save your life. It is never over until it's over. I learned that my body is resilient. I transformed my body from dumpy, achy and slow to one that is sleek, thin and highly energized. It is like going from a Volkswagen Bug to a Ferrari! I knew I wanted to be fit, I just never thought in my wildest dreams that I could be where I am at now. Once again, if I can do it, anybody can. I will also add that it doesn't matter what your age or health status, it is never too late to change your life for the better.

The value is looking at the big picture of life, and not in strictly losing weight for vanity purposes. Let's face it, we are all vain, but as time went on I realized I was taking responsibility for my life. I was taking ownership of the state of my health. My morbidity, that part of my life when my body will eventually fail, will be a tiny sliver of time, hopefully, happening at the very end. I want to spend as little time in doctor's offices and hospital waiting rooms as possible. This is where the real value is as far as I am concerned. It is up to us to take care of our bodies so that we will be strong, flexible and healthy for long as possible. Working your body hard with free weights, eating right and doing cardio exercises will build new muscle tissue and bone matrix. Looking good is fine, but looking good and being healthy is fantastic. We need to keep growing both physically and mentally. We are worth it!

The years 2012-2013 were time well spent. I achieved my goals of losing weight and becoming super fit. I loved the journey and what it took to get to where I am now. I hope I live well into old age. And if I don't, it won't be for lack of trying. Not only was this time well spent, but I can now say it was time spent well.

Epilogue

"Believe you can and you're halfway there."

—Theodore Roosevelt

As I write this, I am coming up to my one-year anniversary of reaching my goal weight of 110 pounds. In other words, I have maintained my weight for almost a full year. This is no small achievement. I would rank maintaining my weight right up there with losing it. When you are in losing mode you have your eye on the prize—your goal weight. Maintenance is a life-long endeavor. It is also a daily management activity involving counting calories in and calories out. I have logged into the online food journal that I use, My Fitness Pal, for over 650 days in a row. It is a way of life. It is also a way of keeping score.

I have accepted the fact that I can no longer eat with abandon. I have trained myself to think in terms of how many calories are in the foods I eat and how many calories I burned during my workouts. Logging in keeps me accountable and informed. This is the formula for my success. I stay within my daily-allotted calorie number of 1590. My average burn through exercise is 600 - 800 per day. And I eat a lot of food—good food.

I go to the gym six days per week. It is another tool that keeps me slim. The workouts are a combination of cardio and strength training, and they last 70-90 minutes. Some days are better than others. This may sound like a lot, but it is just a part of my day, a very important part. I push myself hard and make my workouts count. I see people day after day, month after month, working out on treadmills, elliptical and arc machines, yet their bodies do not change. I would bet that they are not counting their calories.

I constantly tweak and change different parts of my workouts. My goals these days are to keep changing my body composition to more muscle and less fat. For all those women who think they will turn into Arnold Schwarzenegger if they lift weights, fear not. It takes time and a lot of hard work to build up muscle tissue. I have muscle definition in my arms and back, which is an awesome feeling at 57 years old. People who are in their fifties and up do not have to look dumpy or have a body composition of bones and fat. In fact, having a healthy, fit and hard body is within reach of everyone if you do the work. Not only will you look good but you will also improve the quality of your life exponentially.

Vanity. I admit that I love being thin and healthy. I love buying clothes in small sizes that fit. Sometimes I still can't believe I weigh 110 pounds. I look in the mirror without fear now. When I walk into a building with reflective glass, I do not turn away. I love not being fat. My mind is still catching up with my new look. Sometimes when I dream at night, I am that overweight person I used to be. Actually, that is a nightmare. This happens less and less. People do treat you differently. Yeah, I know, this is not fair, but it's reality. The fantastic part of this reality is that we have the capability to change it starting right this minute. Change happens in an instant if we want it to. Sometimes it is simply changing our outlook or attitude. For example, sometimes when I am working out it feels like a slog. I press on and say to myself, "I love working out on the Arc machine" over and over. Eventually, my body fatigue catches up with my mind, and I find my rhythm. I make sure to take a rest day each week. I determine when my rest day will be by how I feel that day. This works well for me.

A few weeks ago I had my annual physical. Instead of dreading this appointment like I used to, I was actually looking forward to it. I wanted to see some positive results. My blood pressure (120/68) and cholesterol numbers were excellent. My resting heartbeat of 48 alarmed the health team. I soon found myself hooked up to an EKG machine to make sure everything was okay with my heart. I knew I was just fine, but they were looking at me like I was a 57-year-old woman who had, what they thought was an abnormally low-resting heartbeat. As it turned out, my results were perfect. One of the health technicians asked if I was a runner because I had an "athlete's heart." How cool is that? This incident made my day.

I also had an evaluation of my ankle with Dr. Michael Weaver, the Orthopedic Trauma rock star at Brigham and Women's Hospital. I hadn't seen him in over a year and a half. He said I looked healthy, and he was impressed that I used my accident to change my health and life. Dr. Weaver tells all of his patients to look at their injuries as an opportunity to change their lives in a positive way, whether that be losing weight, quitting smoking or developing a healthier lifestyle. Most people don't take his advice, so it was fun to be one of the few who did. By the way, my ankle with the 11 pins and two plates are doing just fine. The hardware stays.

My energy level is through the roof these days. I am no longer fatigued from carrying an extra 80 pounds around. I get fatigued when I work out. If I can, I try and use my car less, which means more walking. I walk to and from the gym. I walk to the library. I walk to the supermarket. I know; I can hear people saying, "I don't have time to walk places." There is definitely planning involved, but it adds to my calorie burn and keeps me upright and moving. Sitting is bad for my health. I can easily kill an hour online. What a waste of time. I found out that stretching while watching a television show, especially sports, is a great way to stay flexible. I cannot sit for very long anymore and that is a good thing.

As I mentioned earlier, you are treated differently when you are in good shape. I notice this type of behavior more and more, especially when I watch other people. People who are over 50 and overweight are invisible in our youth obsessed society. This isn't going to change. The argument is that we should accept ourselves for who we are and what we look like. This may be true in fairyland. Everyone I know, fat or thin, young or old, wants to look good. When you look good, you give off a positive, confident vibe. This positive energy is infectious and people notice. You are no longer invisible.

The issue of food addiction is at the top of my list these days. If people really thought about their food addictions it would help them understand why they are overweight and also lighten up on the negative self-esteem and self-worth feelings that make us feel awful about ourselves. This awareness is the first step in addressing the issue on how to change our eating habits for life. I still have a mad sugar addiction. My two treat days each month include frosting, cake or ice cream or all three. I couldn't do this anymore often than this. This is just the way I am. Everyone is different. Knowledge adds to our personal power.

A long time ago, I read the wonderful book, *Key To Yourself,* by Venice Bloodworth. It is about self-improvement. Venice believed that that you could choose the age you wanted to be regardless of your actual age. I decided that I would try this theory out for myself. I loved being in my 40s, especially my early 40s. I decided that in my mind I was now 42 even though I am 57. Forty-two was a good time in my life. I was in shape and I had just completed the New York Marathon. I was happy. Over the next twelve years as I gained weight I looked older than my chronological age. I was not happy.

I had lunch with my friend, Mark, recently. Mark is a dear friend and my former photo editor. Mark is 44 years old. He has known me at my peak weight of 190 pounds and has marveled and been supportive during my weight loss endeavor. When I saw him for lunch he said, "You are fitter than the last time I saw you. You look younger; you look to be my age." The theory works! I am only two years off my new age of 42. I was giving off a new, younger, healthier vibe. I may be chronologically 57 years old, but in my mind I am 42! I love it!

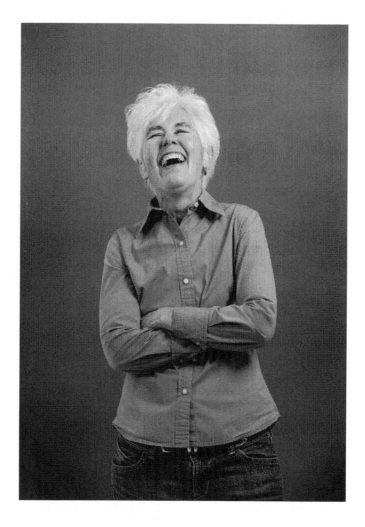

I met a lovely woman—named Mary—recently at my gym. I had just gotten off the Arc Trainer and Mary was getting ready to hop on. We chatted and she mentioned that she had noticed my weight loss progress during the past year. Mary then told me that she had just lost 72 pounds. Her doctor wanted her to lose 20 more but she found herself stuck in plateau mode. I suggested she try counting her calories and pushing a little harder at the gym. A week later Mary came up to me with a big smile on her face. She told me she had upped her level on the Arc Trainer from three to ten and lengthened her workouts from ten to 30 minutes! Impressive. She had also signed on with an online food journal and started counting her calories. The best part was that she was so proud of herself for taking positive action.

It was at this point that I told Mary that I was doing some research for a book I had written and would she agree to a short interview. I interviewed Mary later that evening and learned a lot about her history of struggling with her weight. I asked her if she read my story what value would she like to gain from it. She didn't hesitate. "How did you do it and how did you keep it off?" Mary told me many things, including that she is 67, divorced, and lives alone. Her goal was to live a healthy lifestyle and have an extended healthy aging process because in her words, "My children aren't adding in-law apartments onto their homes any time soon." I loved her honesty and practicality. I believe there are a lot of folks out there who think like Mary.

I have made a pledge to myself that I will always weigh 110 pounds or less for the rest of my life. I affirm this several times per day. Working out and eating right are right up there with showering and brushing my teeth every day. It is my reality and I love it.

I am excited about life. I am over 50, but I am no longer overweight or out of breath. I am super fit. I am doing everything possible to maintain excellent health and make sure I stay this way.

To all of you who think you cannot turn back the clock by losing the weight and getting super fit, please believe me when I say, with all of my heart, that you can. Decide, be positive and go forward. If I can do this, you can too, because I am just like you.

Acknowledgements

Hillary Clinton, love her or hate her, one thing we can all agree upon is the title of one of her books, *It Takes A Village*. It simply means that when creating something special or trying to reach a goal it takes many people, not just one. The creation of this book depended on the talents and good will of many people that I know well and some who I am just beginning to know. I would like to extend my most sincere gratitude to the following individuals.

My good friend and mentor, Dr. Terrence Russell, was instrumental in guiding me along some of the perilous pathways of business. His sage advice kept me on my toes and motivated me to never forget to dream big.

Friends and authors, Bob and Julie Kembel, gave this rookie valuable time and advice about the book publishing process. Editor, Kathy Bremner, took my manuscript and put it through the buzz saw, known as the first editing. Her kindness and diplomatically delivered suggestions helped shape some very raw material into something that could be taken to the next step in the creation process.

I would like to extend my gratitude to the author, Stephen King, for writing the book "On Writing." It is the only book I have read out of the many he has written. He writes in the clear, no nonsense, practical manner only a northern Yankee can offer. He cuts to the chase of what goes into the making of a good read. I highly recommend this book for anyone contemplating writing a book.

I am lucky to have life-long friends who have helped in their own unique way. They are Nancy Souther, Matt Ditullio, Suzanne McCarthy, and my brother, Joey, and I thank them for their valuable input. Also, Alex Jones of Alex Jones Photography. I gave Alex a vision of what I wanted and he delivered in a masterful way.

A special thanks goes out to Mary Kelly, Denise LaPlante, Janie Thompson and Jane Mullin for sharing their stories with me. I would like to also thank my Aunt Mary and Uncle Anthony for inspiring me every day to get up and go to the gym. They are respectively 83 and 86 years old. They go to the gym three times per week and workout hard.

Also, I would like to thank editor/designer, Jean Boles for her excellent skills and service in bringing this book to completion.

Finally, I would like to thank my partner, Linda, for believing in me. It is a wonderful feeling knowing that you have someone in your corner who loves and supports you unconditionally. In the dictionary beside the word kindness is Linda's picture. She is kindness personified. I am the luckiest person in the world.

Sources

Chapter One - #1

Sullivan, J. (2011) Barbell Training is Big Medicine.
Starting Strength.
Retrieved from -
startingstrength.com/index.php/site/barbell_
training_is_big_medicine

Chapter Two - #1

UCLA SNAC (Student Nutrition Awareness Campaign),
SNAC Guide to Nutrition.
Retrieved from - map.ais.ucla.edu/go/1001279

Chapter Eleven - #1

Dickens, C (1843) A Christmas Carol, Tribeca Books

Chapter Eleven - #2

UCLA SNAC (Student Nutrition Awareness Campaign),
SNAC Guide to Nutrition.
Retrieved from - map.ais.ucla.edu/go/1001279

Chapter Thirteen - #1

Centers for Disease Control and Prevention. Adult BMI
Calculator. Retrieved from -
www.cdc.gov/healthyweight/assessing/bmi/adult_bmi
/english_bmi_calculator/bmi_calculator.html

About the Author

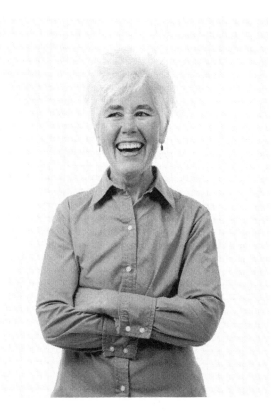

L aura Sinclair is a writer, motivational speaker, and photographer. She lives in the great state of Massachusetts.